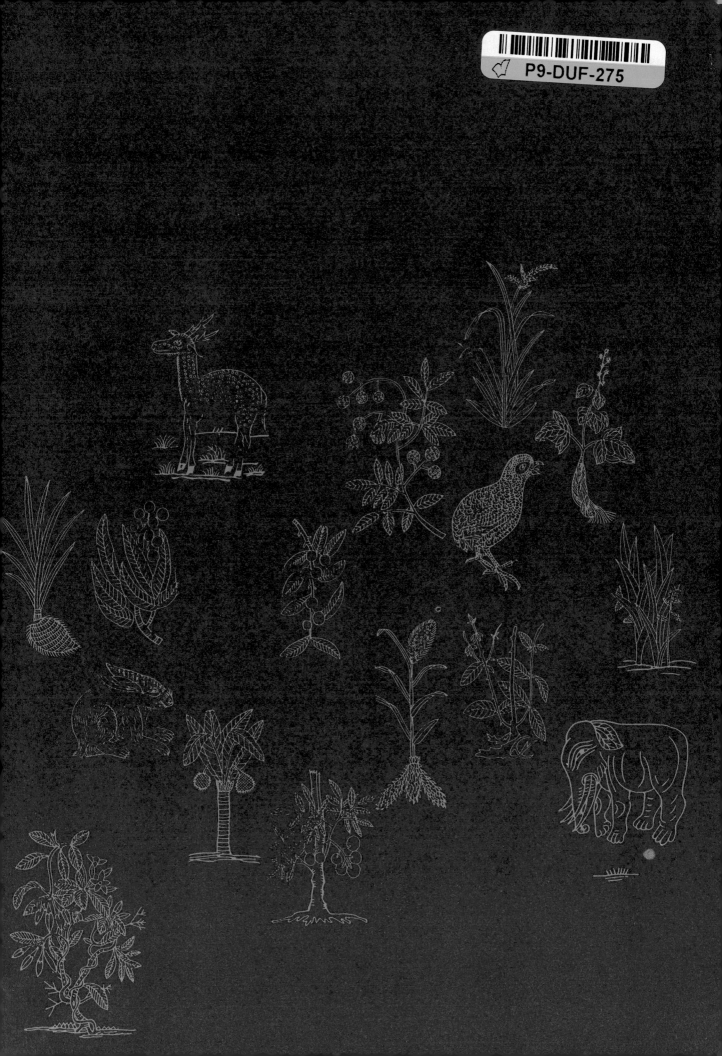

Chinese
Herbal Medicine

Editor-in-Chief: Allan Amsel

Editors: Maureen McClellan
Derek Maitland

Art Direction: Hon Bing-wah

Photography: Nik Wheeler

Botanical drawings: Myumi Terao

Other photo credits: Cover: John Leung;

SHAMBHALA PUBLICATIONS, INC.
HORTICULTURAL HALL
300 MASSACHUSETTS AVENUE
BOSTON, MA 02115

Second Printing 1990

Printed in Korea

Distributed in the United States by
Random House and in Canada by
Random House of Canada Ltd.

ACKNOWLEDGEMENTS

The Publisher is particularly indebted to
Paul But, BSc, MA, CPh, PhD, Curator,
Chinese Medicinal Materials Reserach
Centre, Chinese University of Hong Kong,
for his advice and assistance, also to
Chan Sio Man for her work checking the
Pinyin romanisation of Chinese characters
used in this book.

Library of Congress Cataloging-Publication Data

Reid, Daniel P., 1948–
  Chinese herbal medicine.

  Bibliography: p.
  1. Herbs — Therapeutic use. 2. Materia
medica — China. 3. Medicine, Chinese.
I. Title. RM666.H33R45 1987
615'.321'0951 86-17814
ISBN 0-87773-397-X
ISBN 0-87773-398-8 (pbk.)

Chinese
Herbal Medicine

Daniel P. Reid

SHAMBHALA
Boston
1990

Contents

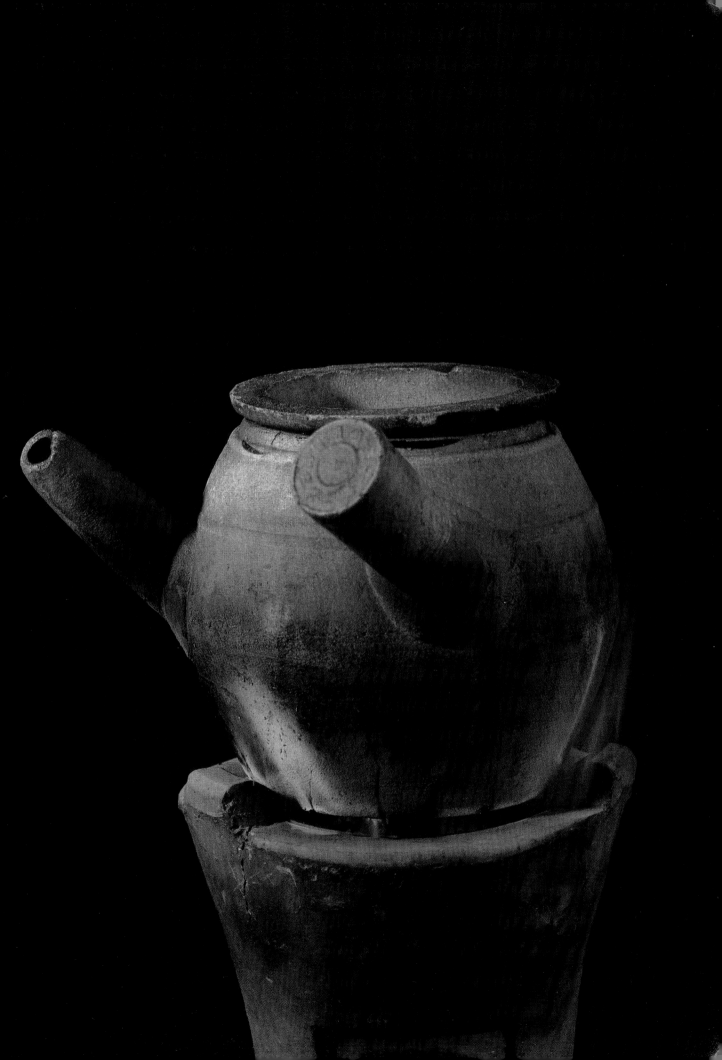

Foreword

The art of practising Chinese herbal
medicine stretches back over more than
5000 years, embracing all the domains
of nature — earth and sea, season and
weather, plant and animals — and all
the elements that constitute the
universe. Contemporary Chinese
medicine represents the cumulative
clinical experience and time-tested
theories of five millenia of continuous
practice by traditional Chinese
physicians. It remains the world's
oldest, safest, and most comprehensive
system of medical care, developing as
dynamically today as throughout its
long history. It seems about time for the
West to start paying serious attention
to Chinese medicine, and to benefit
from its profound insights and potent
remedies. It is towards this end that
Chinese Herbal Medicine was written.

To insure an original and
comprehensive approach to the subject,
all research for the book was done from
original Chinese sources, both ancient
and contemporary. While readers may
find some of the concepts and
terminology somewhat exotic at first, I
hope that the material is presented
clearly enough so that, with a little
further thought, the insights will be
gained. For those who wish to pursue
various aspects of the subject, a brief
bibliography of other available works
in English is provided at the end of the
book.

I owe a special debt of gratitude to
Drs. Huang Powen, Hung Yixiang, and
Sammy J.C. Mei of Taipei, who literally
"showed me the ropes" of Chinese
medicine. Without them, this book
would have been impossible, and it is
to them that it is dedicated.

Daniel P Reid
April 23, 1986
Peitou, Taiwan

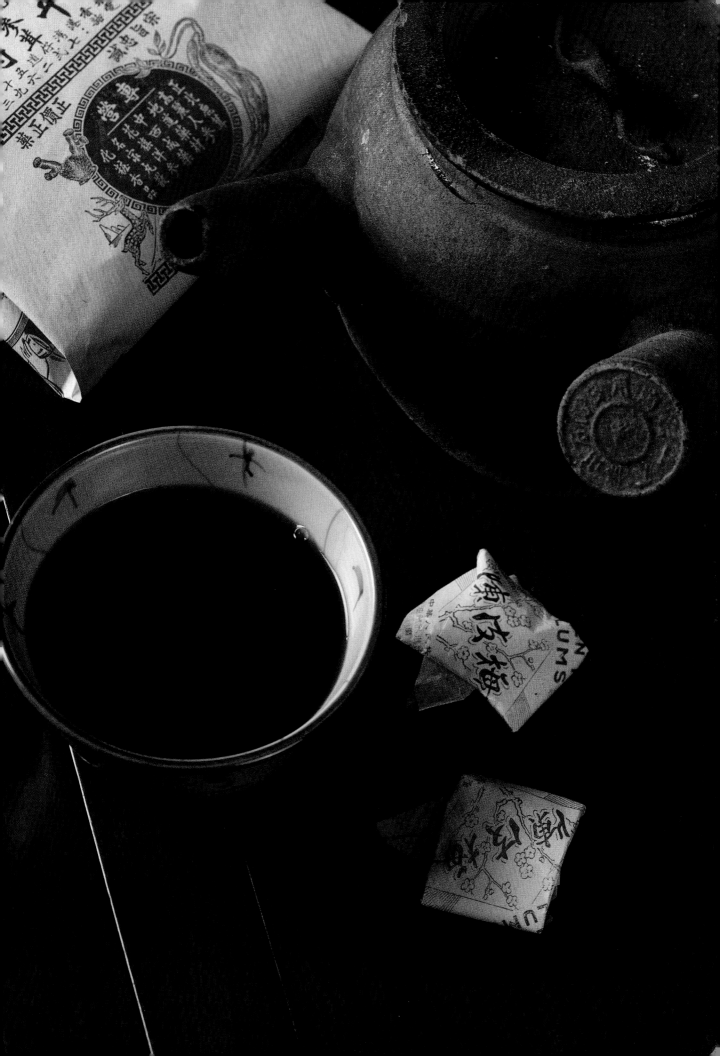

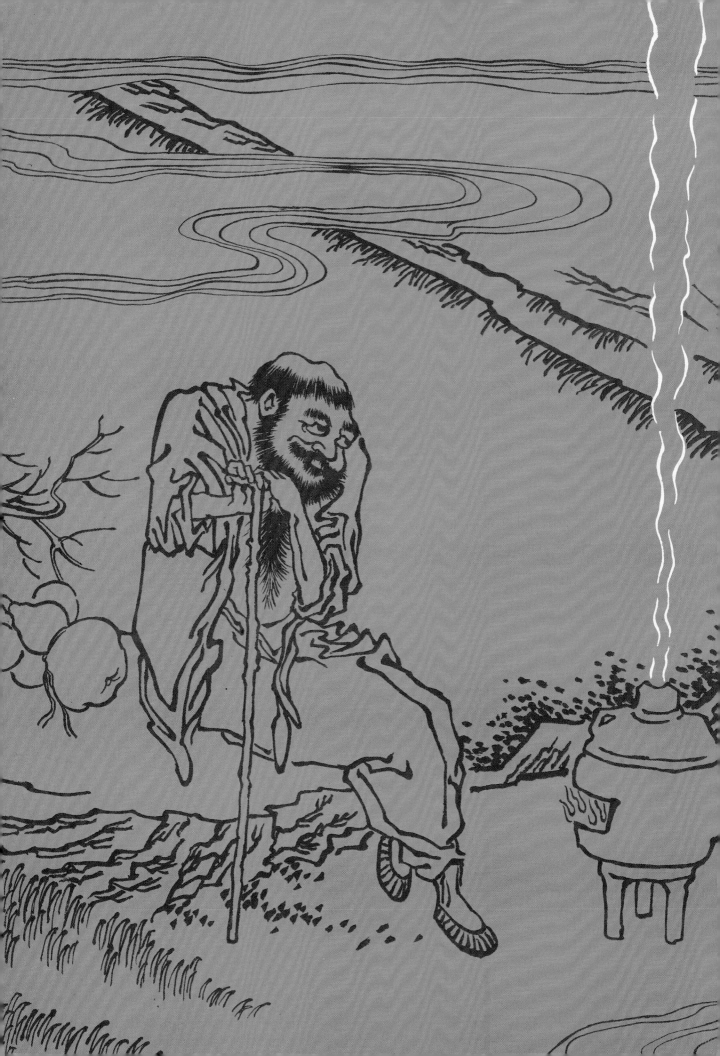

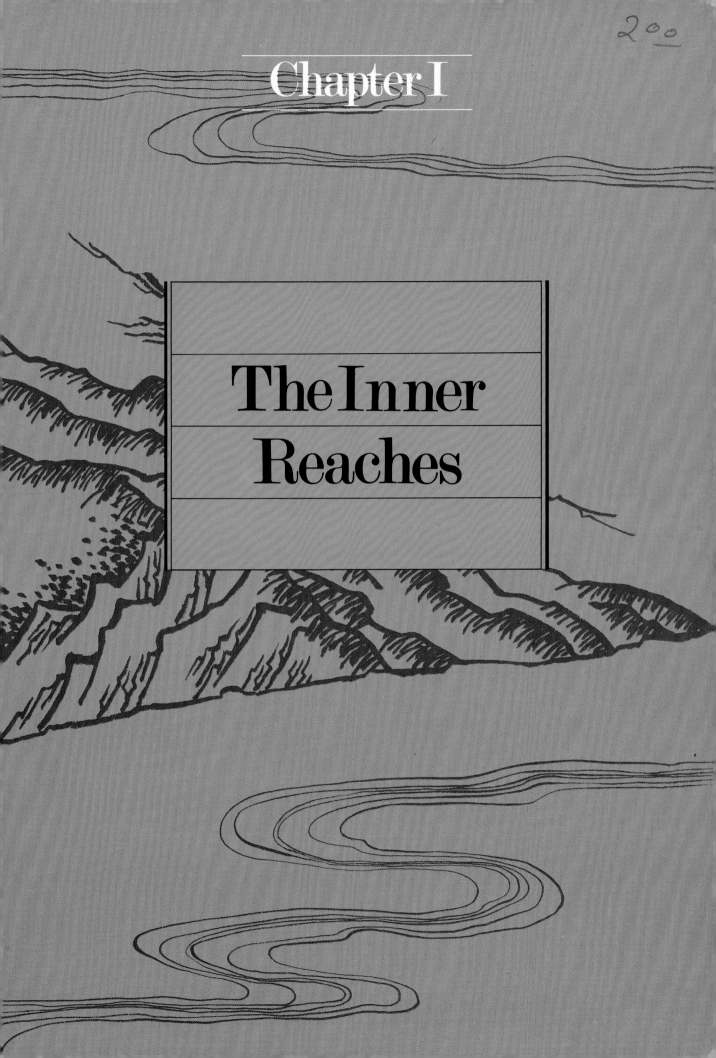

Chapter I

2⁰⁰

The Inner Reaches

any centuries ago, according to Chinese folklore, a farmer in Yunnan found a snake near his hut and beat it senseless with a hoe, leaving it for dead. A few days later he discovered the same snake slithering in his yard, and again he tried to kill it. When the apparently indestructible reptile appeared again a few days later, the farmer gave it another beating, but this time he watched the bleeding snake crawl into a clump of weeds and begin eating them. By the next morning its wounds were healing again, and it was already recovering its vitality.

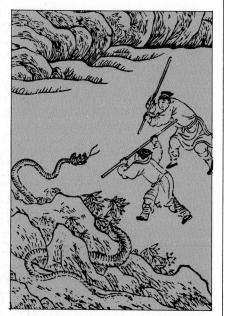

Such was the discovery, as legend has it, of *san qi* (*Panax notoginseng*), the main ingredient of *Yunnan bai yao*, a white herbal powder that counteracts internal or external bleeding. It does this by bonding the edges of wounds and swiftly healing torn tissue. It is also called *shan qi,* meaning "mountain varnish".

It would take more than a little historical licence to suggest that many millions of people have since owed their lives to a lowly, indomitable reptile. Nonetheless, it is known for a fact that the medicinal plant proved to be so effective a treatment for combat wounds over many centuries of military conflict in China that the soldiers paid tribute to its precious qualities by calling it *jin bu huan*, or "gold-no-trade." And it has quite understandably been a powerful, key weapon in the vast arsenal of potions, powders, pills, salves, tonics and other remedies of Chinese herbal medicine.

The same alchemy of myth and fact must be taken into account in any comprehensive study of the roots and growth of Chinese herbal medicine, and the element of myth and folklore is likewise understandable. For just as the developed pharmacopoeia of this medical science is vast, so too is its history, going back at least 5,000 years. Chinese historians attribute the discovery of herbal medicine to a legendary emperor, Shen Nong (3494 B.C.), who is said to have introduced agriculture to his people and to have become fascinated and intrigued by the apparent medicinal properties of various plants. "Shen Nong tested the myriad herbs,"wrote the great Han dynasty historian Sima Qian, "and so the art of medicine was born."

Even then, it was many centuries before myth and fact could begin to be scientifically separated. Within that time there were no written records, save for primitive inscriptions of prayers for the sick carved on pieces of tortoise carapace and animal bones, and the discoveries and remedies of Shen Nong and the shamans and sorcerers of that ancient era were passed from generation to generation by word of mouth. This naturally led to a great deal of superstition and symbolism —treatments and remedies and, indeed, even maladies that we in the West would call "old wive's tales"— and the great storehouse of this science, even as it stands today, is still riddled with herbal, animal and mineral drugs, and various combinations of them, that were selected mainly for their symbolic and emblematic significance rather than proven medicinal properties. This is not to say that Chinese herbal medicine is largely a concoction of quack theories, for within the proven and unproven science of this medical practice there is an essential and long-established element of *faith*—a principle that Western medical science is beginning to turn its attention to today in its bid, through research into placebos, to link technology and psychology into a more "total" form of treatment. And in this context, it could be rash to say that there is absolutely no remedial value at all in stalactites and staghorns as a tonic for the renewal of youthful vigour, in fossil bones and oyster shells as astringents, or verdigris, bear's gall and turtle shell as purgatives—or dried centipedes, scorpions, silkworms and beetles, the exuviae of cicadae, bat's dung, tiger's bones, hedgehog skins, minerals such as realgar, brown mica, cinnabar ore and clay and the myriad herbs, plants and shrubs that form the pharmacopoeia of herbal medicine.

Antiquity and faith built the storehouse of this science, and it is a testament to the power of herbal medicine that all its lore and symbolism has flourished and survived to this day, adding much to its exotic and bizarre nature, if indeed casting a shadow upon its validity as a time-honoured complement or even challenge to modern medicine. Science itself is now vigorously testing that validity, and with some interesting results. In 1983, for example, public health officials in Beijing announced that a 400-year-old prescription for the treatment of hemorrhoids had been tested on 40,000 patients has proved to be 96-percent effective and had been officially designated as a cure. They described the remedy as "an injection of insect secretions on sumac leaves mixed with crystal salt."

But certainly, it can safely be imagined that in the mists of its beginning Chinese herbal medicine developed at the flickering evolution of fact and fiction, of sorcery and superstition and peasant wisdom. If we accept that the emperor Shen Nong was the father of this science, then we must appreciate that it was probably another 2,000 years before the herbal observations attributed to him and to others who followed him were actually committed to writing. It took that long, as well, for the very concept of medicine to take its place in the Chinese written language— medicine as *yao* and doctor as *yi*. It was another half-century, about 500 B.C., before the term *ben cao* appeared to describe the concept of herbal medicine and its growing pharmacopoeia—*ben* meaning any plant with a rigid stalk and *cao* any grass-like plant. This term eventually embraced ingredients and medicines taken from the animal and mineral worlds too, and it continues to describe the collective arsenal of herbal medicine today.

It was in this period, about 500 years before the birth of Christ, that the science of herbal medicine was absorbed inextricably as a key element of Chinese philosophy and spiritualism. Its faith, folklore and proven science became an integral part of religious doctrine, and this role in Chinese spiritual life must be understood before an understanding of its own philosophy and technique can be arrived at. Far from being just a form of medical treatment, it is still

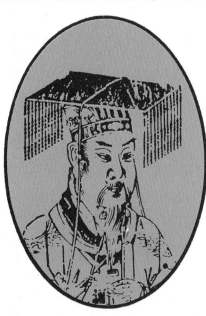

firmly planted at the core of a philosophy that encompasses the well-being of the body and the soul, a code of spiritual and social behaviour and even a compelling and possibly a valid attempt to define the very meaning of life.

The roots of this philosophy are said to go back, again, to the emperor Shen Nong. By some ancient accounts he is said to have not only tested many medicinal herbs but also "wrested from Nature a knowledge of her opposing principles." Over the centuries that followed his reign, Chinese alchemists, geomancers and

OPPOSITE Ancient wood block print depicts climax of a hunt for snakes, an important herbal medicine ingredient. ABOVE Emperor Huang-di, one of three mythical fathers of the Chinese civilisation. RIGHT Block print portrait of Shen Nong, the founder of medicine, and stone rubbing of his agricultural work.

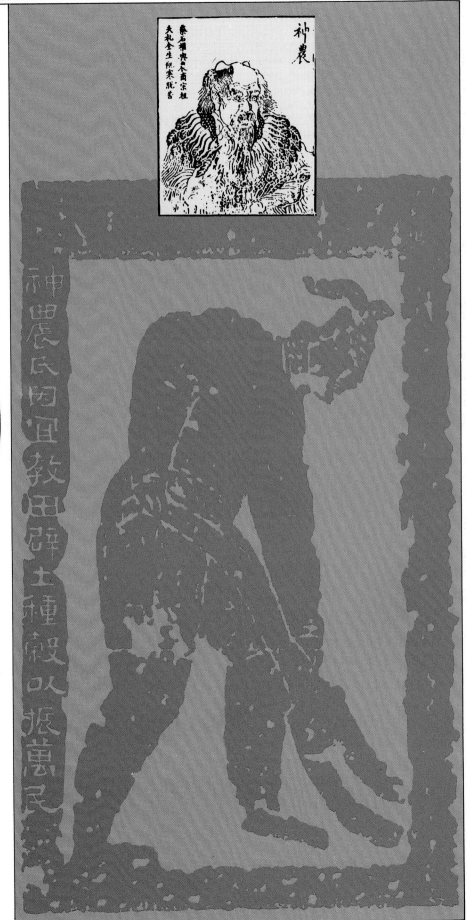

thinkers developed this concept of opposing natural forces into a code by which man could come to terms with the mystery of life and define his own role within that mystery. Shen Nong's "opposing principles" were established as the opposing and yet complementary and reciprocal "yin" and "yang" forces of nature, of all matter, of all action and thought, of all impetus. As a contemporary observation would have it: "Life is an eternal flux, and the universe is the result of the interplay of yin and yang forces, of the dominant and the recessive, the positive and negative."

In the years from about 600 B.C.

to its natural and inevitable fact and pursuing a course of inaction. Never strive nor interfere, he declared, because things would come to a successful conclusion without effort.

It appears that Lao Zi was the man that a whole gamut of Chinese science and philosophy had been waiting for—a convenient symbol and oracle for many of their cherished theories. Certainly they ascribed their own ideas to his teachings, pinning them to the famous figure's obvious prestige, and they deified him as the godhead of a new and uniquely Chinese religion. A new legend eventually established itself in

path the two basic expressions of the Tao lay locked in their perpetual embrace—the positive, active and even aggressive yang, and the negative, passive, receptive yin, their correlation and balance determining the universal order. By the year of 100 B.C., the neo-Confucian thinker, Dong Zhongshu, had refined this philosophy to include the inner reaches of man himself, establishing man as the universe on a small scale, containing within himself the same locked cycle of yin and yang.

It follows then that if physical health became an integral part of the whole body of law of Chinese spiri-

孔子車　孔子也　老子

two giants of Chinese thinking emerged to apply these concepts to a rigid form of belief and personal behaviour. Confucius (551-479 B.C.), celebrated as China's greatest sage, established a code of rules and ethics which began with the premise that there is a right order and harmony to the universe, based upon a delicate balance of yin and yang forces, and that the force exerted by man must be essentially moral. Man, he declared, must cultivate the Five Virtues of benevolence, justice, propriety, wisdom and sincerity in order to exert his own force in this eternal cycle of good and evil.

The teachings of Confucius were echoed by another great sage of that era, Lao Zi, the reputed father of Taoism. Taking the Confucian doctrine of universal order, Lao Zi taught that man himself can only achieve personal harmony by bowing

his name: Lao Zi had been carried in his mother's womb for eighty years, it preached, and was therefore born with white hair. Hence this name, which means "Old Boy." Legend inevitably tampered with Lao Zi's teachings and opinions as well. Despite his code of inaction in the face of a natural order of things, Taoists invented a path to salvation and a spiritual destination—a mythical "Island of the Eastern Sea" where there existed a herb with the power to bestow immortality.

But aside from its mythical aspects, Taoism essentially dealt with the theory of a cosmic law and structure—and man's place within that structure—that Chinese thinkers had been preoccupied with since Shen Nong's "opposing principles." The Tao became the way, or path, within the meaning, right order and universal harmony of being. Along that

tual and social life, the same Taoist principles of correlation and balance of forces applied as well to diet and medicine. Accordingly, food was taken not just for sustenance and survival but also to constantly balance, regulate and tune up both physical and mental health. Food and medicine became interrelated: foods were chosen as much for their therapeutic qualities as for nourishment and taste. They were to be taken in moderation and adjusted to one's state of health. They were categorised according to the nature of their therapeutic value—"cold" foods such as fruit and vegetables, sliced pork, crab and fish recommended to reduce "heat" in the body; "hot" high-protein foods such as fatty meats, eggs, fried and spiced foods and ingredients soaked in wine, taken to heat up and invigorate the system; and then there were "supplementary" foods, also rich in protein and mainly the internal organs of animals (liver, heart, kidney, brains, placenta, penis and uterus), that were taken as an additional tonic and to strengthen the corresponding organ in the human body.

From here, diet and medicine began to merge into more powerful medicinal diets, beginning with herbal tonic of garlic, ginseng or ginger soaked in liquor, then herbal soups to cure mild ailments — salted fish-heads with tofu and ginger to counteract fever or palpitation, or lotus root, daikon radish or watercress soup in pork broth to ward off bronchial infection and colds — then direct medicinal foods, including recipes of loofah, fennel, arrowroot starch or other herbs and plants, to combat the more serious illnesses, skin diseases, allergies and blood poisoning. At each step of this escalating assault on debilitation and ill-health, the paramount concern was the balancing of opposing forces within the metabolism, forces which were inevitably part of the crucial interplay of yin and yang. It was written as early as the reign of Emperor Shen Nong that to keep these forces in harmony "is the duty of the physician, and to restore the equilibrium, when any of them is in excess or deficiency, is the main object of his endeavours."

Some 4,300 years later, in the early part of the 13th century, the physician's duty had not essentially changed. "Physicians," declared one expert of the time, "must first recognise the causes of an illness and know that transgression of the normal (balance of yin and yang) has taken place. To correct this imbalance, adequate diet is the first necessity. Only when this has failed should drugs be prescribed." And it was here, it can be said, that the full force of a 5,000-year-old folk-science came into play.

There are many examples and detailed descriptions in Chinese literature of the herbal physician at work. And one major point that emerges from these texts is an imperishable tradition, and one that not only explains a great deal about the science itself but also anticipates its latter-day relationship with contemporary Western medicine — and,

indeed, the fate that was to befall the entire traditional culture of China by the turn of the twentieth century. Put in its simplest terms, tradition died hard in Old China, and tradition ultimately brought about its downfall. This apocalyptic cultural collapse in the floodwave of modern Western influence was superbly chronicled by the writer Lin Yutang in 1939 in the novel *Moment in Peking*, an epic story of China in the throes of violent change. Lin Yutang's novel not only explained the influences that brought about this relatively sudden and catastrophic sweeping away of Chinese tradition, it also showed quite graphically the tenacity with which one of the key traditions, herbal medicine, had continued to flourish right up to the advent of this century, with all its practices and beliefs intact. Vast as the practice of herbal medicine was, it faced doom in the struggle with modern Western medical techniques.

In *Moment in Peking*, the eldest son of a prominent Mandarin's family had contracted a serious intestinal fever known as "shang han," "the most dreaded, the most debated, the most written about, the most obscure and the least understood, and the most complicated disease in Chinese medicine." The time of this tragedy was shortly after the Boxer Rebellion of 1900, when the British expeditionary force in China was pressing hard on the tottering Manchu rule and when Chinese science and philosophy, and the empire's entire social fabric, were being torn apart by an incoming flood of Western technology, physics and chemistry, mathematics, astronomy and geography — and medicine.

At first, the condition of the young heir, Pingya, appeared to have improved "by his drinking a medicinal stew of sickle-leaved hare's ear and other plants much relied upon for all kinds of colds, and when he was convalescent he had pills made of various ingredients from cardamom, Sichuan varnish and nutgrass, which drove off the illness definitely." But he was weak, and his system vulnerable, and within weeks he was ill again. This time, the aid of the Imperial Physician was sought, and he prescribed a stew of ephedra,

cinnamon barks, fried licorice powder and almonds to induce perspiration. It was now fairly certain that Pingya had in fact fallen victim to the dreaded *shang han*, and now the physician's attention turned to the crucial physiological forces which, according to tradition, had to be balanced in order to restore the young man's inner harmony.

The disease was "supposed to attack first the three yang systems, and might pass on to any of the three yin systems or all three. The three yang systems are regarded as the alimentary or nourishing systems, being the small intestine, the large

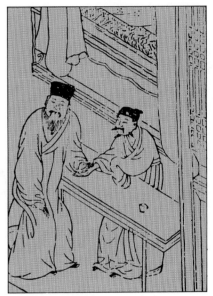

intestine, and the entrances to the stomach, the bladder and the pylorus; at times we speak of the 'six yang systems' including the bladder, the gall-bladder and the stomach. The lungs, the heart, and the membranes around the heart with the pancreas, the kidneys, and the liver, form the yin group, responsible for respiration, circulation and elimination. The terms yin and yang are regarded as relative and complementary, and not as absolute and mutually exclusive. The nourishing systems (yang) support and build up body heat and strength while the other exchange systems (yin) regulate and secrete liquids for lubricating the body. the kidney, the liver, and the

OPPOSITE Stone rubbings of the carriage of Confucius and the renowned sage meeting Laozi, the founder of Taoism. ABOVE The patient's pulse was recognised as a key to diagnosis and health from the earliest stages of Chinese herbal medicine.

13

pancreas in particular are regarded as secreting important fluids for balancing the system."

Pingya's condition grew worse. His fever ran high, his pulse was weak, he began vomiting, his limbs were cold and he complained of a "cold pain" in the abdomen, which was tender and full. "By all signs, the yang systems had 'collapsed within' and the disease had spread to the yin systems. It seemed that his body was being dried up, and his throat became parched and his eyes dull. The doctor no longer tried to 'bring out' the fever by ephedrine and cinnamon bark and licorice, but recognised the necessity of 'concili-atory medicine' to tone up or 'warm up' the yin systems, for it was now recognised that it was a kind of yin cold and the secreting organs were not functioning properly. For this, a stew of autumn roots, dried ginger, the white of small onions and pig's gall were used. Then, as the patient grew steadily worse, a more drastic medicine was used, consisting of rhubarb, thorny limebush, *magnolia officinalis* and even *mangxiao*, a product of saltpeter in fine crystals."

Desperate now, Pingya's parents hurriedly arranged for him to be married, hoping that love and the tender care of his bride would breathe new strength into him. Meanwhile, he was prescribed regular tonics of hot silver fungus in

chicken soup, and when these failed to help him the physician turned to the "Big Sustaining Stew" which, Lin Yutang explained, was used for "at-tacking organic or substantial fever, which differs from functional fever. Every illness comes from the disturb-ance of some vital force and is only brought on by some external cold or heat. It is like a plant; if the root is strong some branches will prosper, and if the root is affected the branches dry up."

But the use of saltpeter, an ingredient of gunpowder, signalled that Pingya's condition was probably already beyond hope. "It is used only for substantial fever in the blood, and then only in extreme cases, to remedy dry heat in the body and soften hard formations. It is so powerful that it softens metals and dissolves stones. When there is sub-stantial fever you have to clean the blood with it. But it must be used sparingly, otherwise it injures the system. When there is poison in the body, the poison receives the effect of the purgative, but if there is no poison then the bodily system itself is injured." In the end, even this extreme antidote could not save the young man. Within days of his hast-ily-arranged wedding, he was dead.

Within a matter of a few years, Chinese medical science—certainly at the level of the wealthier and middle-class Chinese—was engulfed and relegated to a secondary role by Western medicine. It was usurped not because its theories and treat-ments were necessarily redundant, or wrong, or disreputable, but because of a basic philosophical difference between the two practices. In the religion of thought and action that encompassed herbal medicine, the thrust of the medicine itself was toward preventive care—often a long and ponderous study of all aspects of a patient's condition, physical and mental, ancestral, and even environ-mental. Chinese physicians tended to reject the idea of instant remedies, believing that most illness and debili-tation were the result of deep-rooted problems and that without contin-uous long-range treatment the root-problem would simply manifest itself again and again, in different forms and in different parts of the body.

Twentieth century Western medi-

cine, on the other hand, brought with it the art of surgery, more ad-vanced drugs and techniques aimed at the relatively swift cure of the immediate problem. A much wider cultural challenge had to be taken into account as well. In the early centuries, and indeed right into the golden Ming dynasty of the 1600s, Chinese science and technology—and that, of course, included its medical science—had been some 1,000 years ahead of developments in the West. By the turn of this century, however, the Western nations had accomplished a remarkably swift technological and scientific boom, far outstripping the Chinese sciences, which had languished and stultified under the closed and insular influ-ences and restrictions of the Manchu Qing dynasty. Now, as this last of the great dynasties collapsed, any-thing Western was seized upon by a large part of the educated Chinese population, mainly the young, in what was to become the birth of a long and painful, and sometimes violent campaign to redress the arrogant failure of the Manchu reign and catapult China into the modern world.

Yet the science of herbal medicine was not swept away in this, the first of many Chinese cultural revolutions. It survived, and it did this because its philosophy and tradition were so deeply ingrained in the Chinese psy-che, especially that of the landed masses; because its concept of pre-ventive care and "total" treatment was still so valid, even in the face of apparent Western miracles, that it could not in all conscience be dis-missed; because it was so deeply in-terrelated with diet that, far from being vanquished, it held its ground as a complement and even a vital backup to Western medicine. Thou-sands of traditional Chinese herbal medicine shops in China itsself, Hong Kong, Taiwan, Singapore and any large centre of Chinese settle-ment around the world will testify to this even in this present day. And it may well turn out that in the future the world will be thankful for it.

For all its myth, legend and sym-bolism, herbal medicine is now re-asserting its power, its validity and, in many respects, the triumph of its folk-wisdom. Modern research is

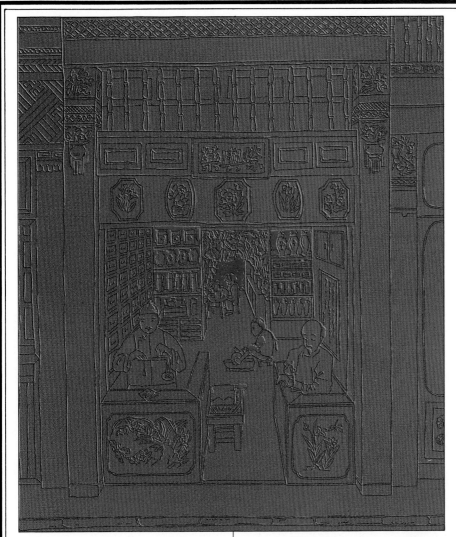

Western medicine is taking a new look at faith-healing in research into the theory and effect of placebos and the psychology of health care. In the United States, the implications of over-specialisation, and its cost, have led to a campaign to bring back the traditional family physician, with his or her more intimate and long-standing knowledge of the patient's emotional and medical needs. Mid-wifery is being restored to take its place alongside the physician. The family environment is being recognised as an important element in health care, removing much of it from the clinical isolation of hospitals. Western medicine, particularly in the United States, is also becoming increasingly concerned about the cost-effectiveness of high-tech medical treatment, and the alarming failure rate of electronic diagnosis. And finally, herbal medicine itself is being promoted as a direct challenge to surgical and clinical science by the emerging field of treatment called "alternative medicine."

It would be presumptuous, and even dangerous, to suggest that either Chinese herbal medicine or Western medicine are superior in their own right. Each have their strengths, and each their weaknesses—herbal medicine still has a great history of symbolism and hidebound tradition to unravel and test, and possibly discard; Western medicine, with its powerful drugs, its medicine and its propensity for the surgeon's knife, must yet come to terms with the consequences of a science that is losing touch with the essential human factor of medical treatment. It would be more realistic by far to suggest that if there was ever a field for a momentous meeting of East and West, it is in the field of medicine— Western medical technology combined with Chinese medical philosophy and herbal treatment; a meeting of future and past, laying the foundation for a new age of medical care in which the eyes of modern electronics and the intuition of a 5,000-year-old science probe together the inner reaches of the human condition.

finally separating its myth and science, and the science is standing up well to the test. It is recognised, for instance, that while the use of anaesthetics in surgery was first introduced in the West in 1847, the Chinese were using "narcotic soups" for minor surgery some 700 years ago. Their use of arsenic and calomel for the treatment of venereal diseases foreshadowed Western practices by at least 400 years. For centuries, the Chinese treated "ulcer of the lung," or streptococcual diseases, with the fermented brine of salted vegetables—a process and remedy similar to modern penicillin. The use of ephedra for the treatment of asthma, established in Chinese medicine as long ago as the second century, has been a Western and world-wide practice only since 1887. Iodine was used by the Chinese at least 1,000 years ago to treat enlarged thyroids; it is now a common remedy in Western medicine. In fact, of the more than 700 drugs applied over the centuries by the Chinese herbal physician, more than 100 have already been tested, and their curative properties confirmed, by modern science.

At the same time, Western medicine, having advanced so rapidly and having rushed almost headlong into specialisation and technology, is now braking and turning much of its attention back toward its own folk-origins. The concepts of preventive care and "total" treatment, traditional in Chinese medicine, are being recognised as integral and important elements of a comprehensive public health and fitness campaign now being launched in the West. Diet, too, has become the catchword of societies alarmed at deteriorating food and health standards in their urbanised, industrialised and stress-oriented environments. "You are what you eat" is Madison Avenue's belated echo of an ancient Chinese wisdom.

OPPOSITE Li of the Iron Crutch, one of the Eight Immortals, or fairies, of Chinese mythology, is often a patron symbol of herbal druggists. ABOVE Block print of a typical druggist's store.

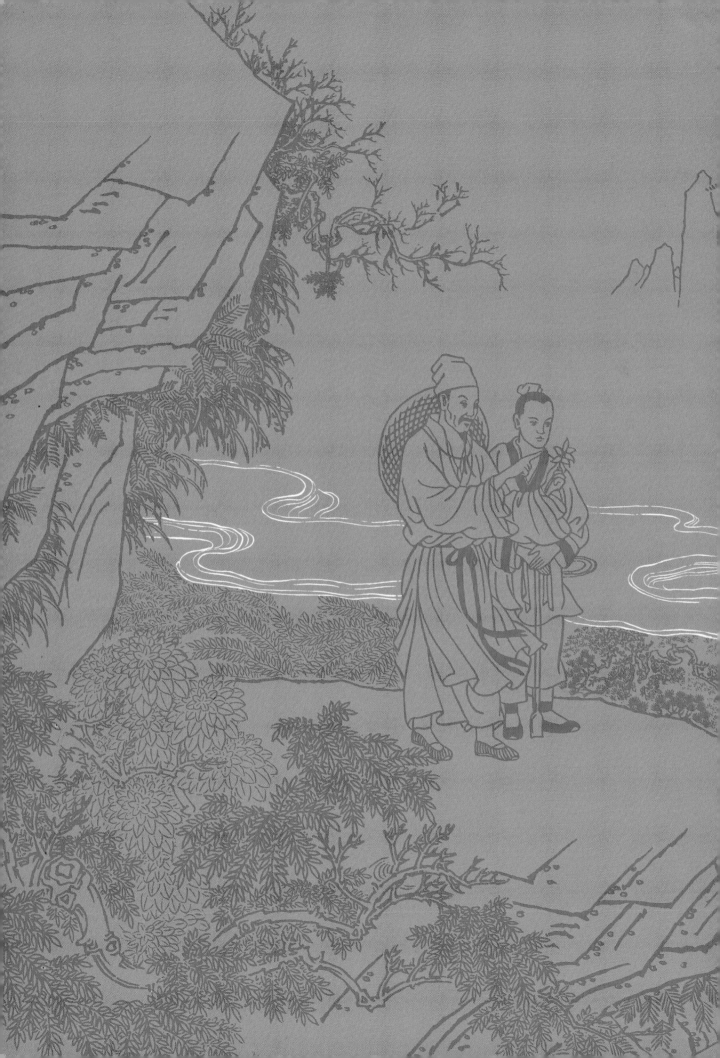

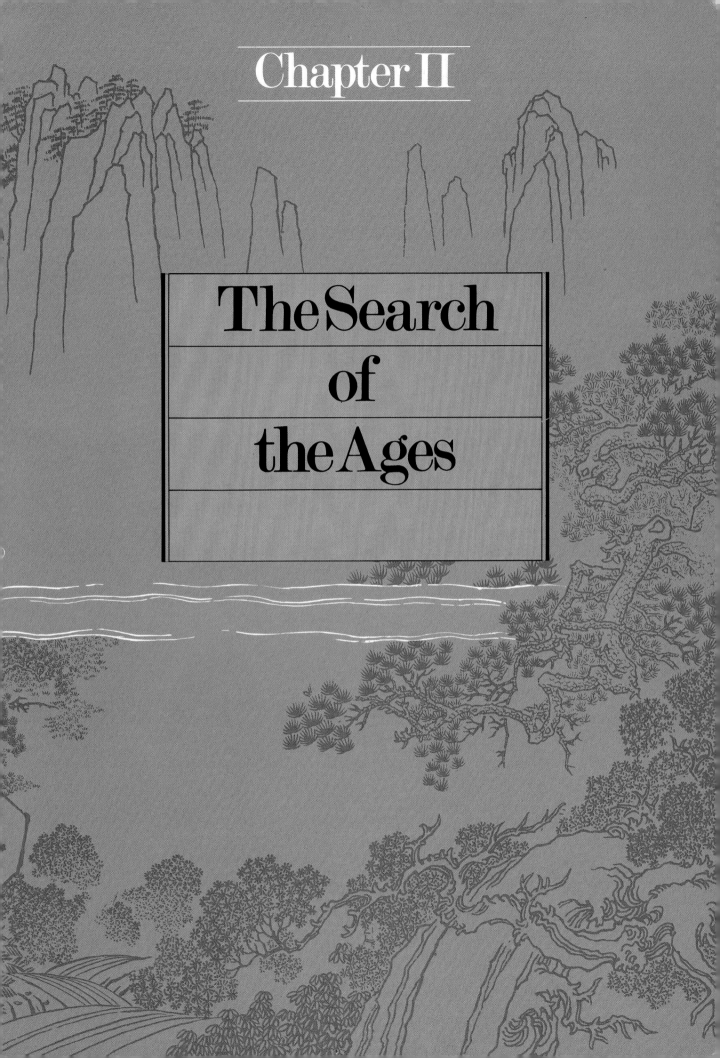

Chapter II

The Search of the Ages

If we were to search for the point in history at which Chinese medicine became a profession—emerging from the hearthside to enter the realm of science—that point is probably the time of the Han dynasty, more than 2,000 years ago. By then a widespread system of orderly government had been established—thus the foundations of Chinese civilisation had been laid—and the Han dynasty was to see this cultural unity become so firmly implanted that it has survived as such to this present day.

More important, from the point of view of this book, is that the keeping of historical records was systemised during the Han period (206 B.C. to A.D. 220). The first steps were taken to record the pharmacopoeia and remedies of herbal medicine, and it is recognised now, from Han relics discovered in Gansu province, that for the educated Chinese at least medical treatment had become an established and relatively sophisticated practice. A subject of the Han reign who felt ill or off-colour could readily refer to what we would regard today as handy booklets giving remedies for specific sicknesses; but these were not books as we know them, they were bamboo or wood strips, as many as 35 of them, bound together with twine, with each strip inscribed with a prescription and recommended dosage. The Gansu "books" include another interesting note: veterinary science had also emerged by this time, for on one strip there is a prescription for treating a horse.

But long before these early records appeared, and long before the initial structure of Chinese civilisation took shape, herbal medicine was claiming a prominent place in the primitive cycle of Chinese tribal life. We speak of a birth whose time we can only roughly establish at around 3500 B.C., and in peering backward into that distant mystery it is difficult to escape the visual cliché of the "mists of time." But in fact the infancy, if not the birth, of Chinese medicine probably was shrouded in mountain mists.

Before the advent of professional physicians, herbal medicine was the domain of tribal shamans, or "medi-

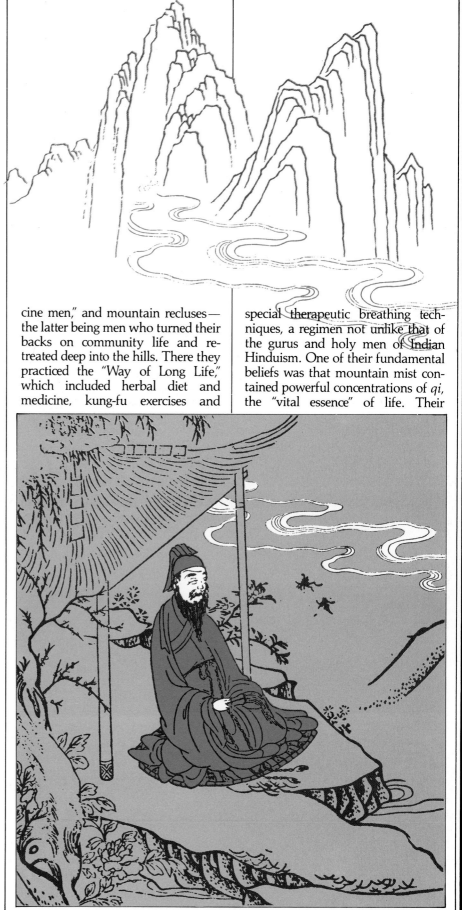

cine men," and mountain recluses—the latter being men who turned their backs on community life and retreated deep into the hills. There they practiced the "Way of Long Life," which included herbal diet and medicine, kung-fu exercises and special therapeutic breathing techniques, a regimen not unlike that of the gurus and holy men of Indian Hinduism. One of their fundamental beliefs was that mountain mist contained powerful concentrations of *qi*, the "vital essence" of life. Their

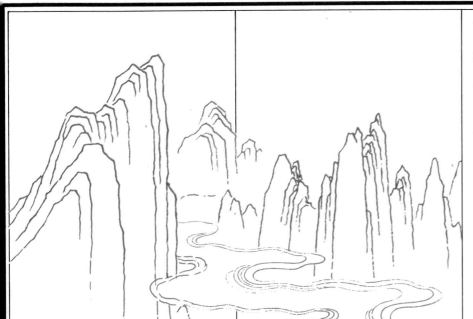

contribution to Chinese medicine was not only the gathering of wild plants and herbs, which they believed to have properties that would nurture, strengthen and prolong life, but also the abiding link between medicine and the martial arts—a link that is kept intact today by certain martial arts masters.

By the time of the Yin dynasty of about 1500 B.C., references to herbal medicine were appearing on oracle bones—inscriptions that are able to give us some insight into the sicknesses and diseases of that time. Some 160,000 inscribed carapaces and bones have been unearthed in archaeological excavations, and a study of them has pinpointed 36 different illnesses that were prevalent among the people of Yin. Also, in this era, medicine was already making its way down from the mountain mists and into the market place. As tribal communities gathered at certain times of the year for seasonal celebrations, rituals and barter, the mountain men descended from their eyries to display their kung-fu skills and trade their herbs and plants for tools, cloth and wine. It was left to the tribal shamans to test the herbs and confirm their medicinal value. It was during this time that the emperor Shen Nong is said to have carried out his own herbal experiments—the first of many Chinese rulers to become avid patrons, and recipients, of the science.

During the ensuing Zhou dynasty,

beginning in 1122 B.C., the written language underwent rapid development, and medicine began to detach itself from the sorcery that had been part and parcel of its heritage. Up until this time the written character *wu*, with its root symbol meaning "sorcery," described the shaman. Now, the bottom portion of the character was changed to the symbol meaning "wine", and the character that now appeared was *yi*, or doctor. This connection between wine and doctor was significant—the Chinese learned to ferment wine from rice, fruits and vegetables very early in their history, and the liquor was used as a base for the concoction and ingestion of herbal medicines. It was found that the alcohol drew out the potent elements in dried herbs, diluted some medicines that were considered too powerful to be taken on their own, aided rapid absorption of the medicine into the bloodstream and, of course, added to the stimulative property of the potion. A well known tonic for nursing mothers, still used in southern China, was simmered fresh chicken, pork, ginger, wood fungus and rice wine or whisky. Some wines were fermented directly from medicinal plants and were called *chang*, a character which made its debut at about the same time as *yi*. The word for medicine itself, *yao*, also first appeared during the early Zhou dynasty. It was formed with the "grass" radical on top of the character, reflecting its original meaning which was "grasses

which cure disease."

The word *yao* appears often in the great Zhou literary classics such as the *Book of Odes*, *Book of History* and *Book of Changes*. In the *Book of Odes*, for example, there are numerous poems which describe maidens plucking medicinal plants in the fields or by rivers. The herbs that they picked were usually prepared as a single remedy, boiled as medicinal soups, but during the last two tumultuous centuries of Zhou rule, referred to as the Spring and Autumn and Warring States period of Chinese history, herbal medicine became more sophisticated, with potions developed from combinations of herbs and plants.

This was a period of turmoil and instability, with feudal lords plotting and warring for power. But it was also a period of great intellectual growth which came about because many learned men simply abandoned society, with its dangers, corruption and intrigue, followed the example of their forebears, the

recluses, and went back to the safety and isolation of the mountains. There, these *xian*, or "Immortals of the Mountains," also continued the traditions of the recluses, experimenting with medicinal herbs; but their goal was more than just everyday health, it was nothing less than immortality—the elusive Elixir of Life. And their search was to become one of the prime driving forces behind much of the development of herbal medicine.

OPPOSITE Shamans or mountain mystics, were the earliest exponents of traditional Chinese medicine. ABOVE A battle chariot of the Warring States period (450-221 BC), when herbal medicine graduated from sorcery to sophistication.

This search obsessed not only the mountain sages but the Chinese aristocracy too. Emperors and feudal barons began sponsoring herbal research projects, and several rulers, grasping for the keys to longevity, actually died after taking concoctions dreamed up by their medical advisers. During the later Han dynasty and the infancy of Taoism, an emperor organised and funded an expedition to locate the Taoist "Island of the Eastern Sea" where it was believed the herb of immortality grew.

If the Zhou dynasty gave medicine its theoretical framework and its status in the language and culture, the science met its first real test in the ensuing Qin dynasty, established by powerful invaders who swept down from the northwest of China. The Qins crushed the warring fiefdoms and set up a stable, centralised bureaucracy that formed the basis of what was to become the Chinese empire. To consolidate his authority and break the mould of the past, the first Qin emperor engineered what was possibly the first of many "cultural revolutions" in Chinese history: he ordered that all the society's books be burned. Almost all. Only books on three subjects were to be withheld from the flames, he decreed — divination, agriculture and medicine.

The Qin dynasty was a short-lived one, lasting only 15 years, but the seeds of civilisation that it planted and nurtured were to begin blooming under the next rulers of China, the Hans. The great Han dynasty was to last nearly four and a half centuries, and it was to become such a vital force in the history of China that the Chinese have since referred to themselves as the "people of Han." Such was the energy of the times that arts, sciences, philosophy and all the other trappings of civilisation flourished. This was the era of Confucius; it was also the spiritual crucible that produced Taoism, along with an even more vigorous study and development of medicine. Under Taoist doctrine the search continued for the fabled Elixir of Life; experimentation with herbal medicines became more and more sophisticated; alchemists and herbalists became prominent figures in the imperial courts, generously funded and no doubt anx-

iously consulted by omnipotent but mortal rulers whose "mandate from heaven," could ultimately be affirmed, it can be said, only by immortality.

One of the emerging Taoist medical doctrines that particularly intrigued these all-powerful and yet politically vulnerable despots was a close association of medicine and sex. The Taoist physicians believed that one of the paths to strength and longevity lay in frequent and prolonged sexual intercourse — a practice that the emperors and nobles could pay wholesale devotion to, con-

sidering the large harems of concubines that they supported.

Taoist theory dictated that while regular and even abandoned sex was good for the health, it had to be accomplished without release of the semen to promote and nourish the vigour of the male. Even at the bed-pillow, the principle of "opposing forces" held sway.

Men were yang, and women yin, and it was considered crucial that in the sexual union of the two the male must retain and conserve his vital and limited yang while absorbing as much as he could of the female's unlimited supplies of yin essence. "If (one) regards sperm as precious and does not ejaculate," it was written, "then life will never be exhausting." Another early sexual manual, referring to the apparently inexhaustible powers of Emperor Huang Di, recounted that "the Yellow Emperor had sexual intercourse with 1,200 girls and became a god, while nor-

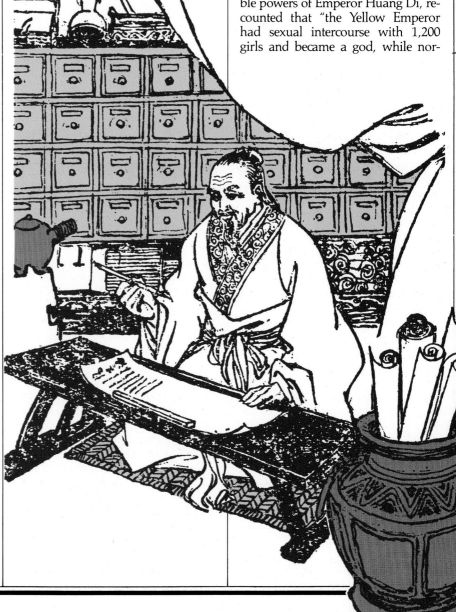

mal people are killed by only one girl ... if one loves the beauty of girls and tries to ejaculate, then his body will be damaged and all kinds of diseases will be encountered. By doing this, one is actually seeking for death." Longevity could be attained, however, by absorbing the female "semen" when she reached orgasm, and at the same time retaining and recycling the male sperm, which was said to travel back up through the male partner's system and nourish the brain.

Medicine played its part in this constant thrust for vitality in the form of herbal tonics which were taken to stimulate sexual potency and to fortify the weaker yang essence of the male. There are many references in the Han era and in later literature to men who had mastered this technique and lived to the age of 150 or more.

On the more mundane level, the expansionist goals of the Han emperors added to the storehouse of herbal medicine. In the conquest of China's fertile southern regions, whole new fields of plants and herbs became available to the herbal scientists and physicians. Other herbs and medicines trickled into the pharmacopoeia by way of trade with India and the Persian Gulf. As the pharmacopoeia grew, the first attempts were made to gather and chronicle the herbal knowledge that had accumulated through the ages. It was during the early Han dynasty that the theories and exploits of the Yellow Emperor were written down in *Huang Di Nei Jing, The Internal Book of Huang Di*. And the attention of the scholars also turned to that other great legendary leader, Shen Nong, recording all herbal knowledge from the time he had "tasted the myriad herbs" to the Han era in a book called *Shen Nong Ben Cao Jing, The Pharmacopoeia of Shen Nong*. In this book all known herbal plants were divided into three categories: an upper class of drugs that nurtured life, a middle group that nurtured "nature" or vitality and a lower group labelled "poisons" or medicines from toxic plants which were used to fight the most virulent diseases.

It is claimed that China's first doctor was Bian Que (407-310 B.C.)

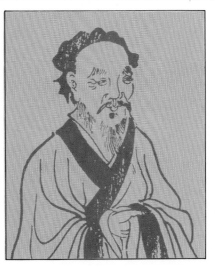

who "practiced medicine and acupuncture and introduced the first gynaecological and pediatrical treatments." If this is true, then China's second most noted physician was almost certainly Dr Zhang Zhongjing who, around 200 B.C., wrote the most celebrated medical treatises of the Han dynasty, *Shang Han Lun*, or *Discussion of Fevers*. More than half of Zhang's family elders are said to have died of fever-related diseases such as typhoid, and he devoted his life to the study of these sicknesses. His book contains 113 medical prescriptions based on 100 medicines, of which more than 80 percent are herbal remedies. One of these is recorded under the name "Cinnamon Sap Soup," prescribed for a variety of chills and fevers, and is a concoction of sap of cinnamon, fresh ginger root, jujubes, licorice root and Chinese peony.

Dr Zhang's book also reflects the continuing study of that time into the yin and yang principles of herbal medicine. He divided diseases into six types, three yang and three yin, and his prescriptions set out to correct imbalances of the two forces by inducing or reducing sweating, elimination or vomiting. He also contributed much to the parallel study of acupuncture by adding the "map" of meridians along which the body's vital energy, or *qi*, was said to flow. It is also known that by the middle of the Han dynasty another book on medicine had appeared, the *Nei Jing*, which included the theory of the circulation of the blood.

It was also during the Han reign that the use of anaesthetics, probably

the first in man's history, appeared in Chinese medicine. It was practiced by another great Han physician, Hua Tuo (A.D. 141-208), who began using herbal "narcotic soups" to numb his patient for the treatment of abcesses, surface tumours and other superficial diseases and wounds. Among the herbal ingredients he used were *Datura metel, Rhododendron sinense* and *Aconitum*. History records that one of the his most noted cases was that of the General Guan Yu, whose arm had been struck in battle by a poisoned arrow. Hua applied his anaesthetic and managed to save the arm, and the general, by scraping away the infected flesh to the bone.

But Hua Tuo was not only a surgeon, he was also a devotee of the early marriage of martial arts and medicine brought about by the mountain recluses; and he developed a series of therapeutic kung-fu exercises based upon the rhythmic movements of five animals, the deer, bear, tiger, monkey and crane. These he prescribed as a regimen to tone up the circulation and respiration, ease constipation and help digestion, limber up the joints, eliminate fatigue and depression and invigorate the heart and kidneys and other vital organs. By the end of the Han dynasty, all the elements that make up what we regard as the "total" treatment of Chinese medicine were firmly in place—its herbal pharmacopoeia, its science, its spiritual beliefs, its sexual code, its therapeutic exercises and its essential relationship with diet. Though there was to be a great deal of experimentation and refinement over the following centuries, these traditions were to reign until the turn of the twentieth century—and, indeed, still govern the science in this present time.

Throughout the Tang, Song and Ming dynasties, therefore, continuing study and practice tended to consolidate the principles of Chinese medicine rather than strike out into new fields of thought. By the beginning of the Tang dynasty (A.D. 608-906) a distinguished herbalist and phar-

OPPOSITE Dr Zhang Zhongjing, the great physician and early scholar of Chinese medicine. ABOVE Bian Que (407-310 BC), claimed to have been China's very first doctor.

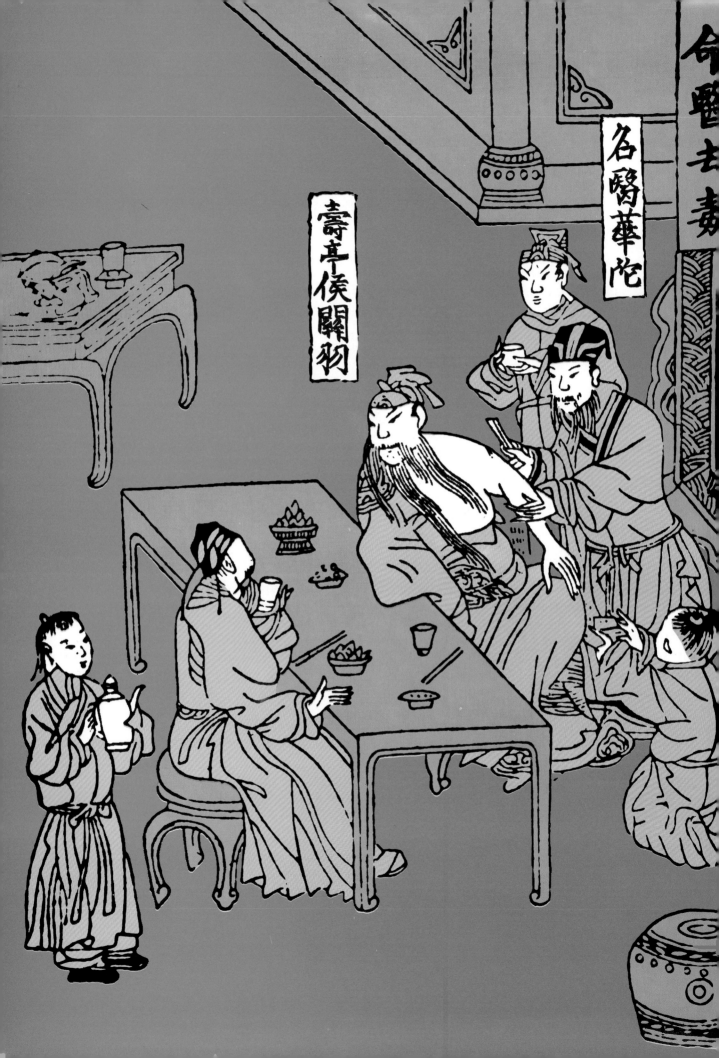

macist, Tao Hongjing, had contributed two new and valuable textbooks to the bibliography of medicine. Once again, the founding discoveries and theories of emperor Shen Nong were echoed, and supported by Dr Tao's own data, in one of these books, *Herbs as Studied by Shen Nong*. The advances made by scholars and physicians since Shen Nong's reign were gathered by Tao and presented in *Anecdotes of Celebrated Doctors*. This process of consolidation was promoted ever further by the founding emperor of the Tang dynasty. He issued a decree that all medical knowledge throughout the empire should be concentrated in the capital, where in A.D. 629 he established China's first school of medicine. Once this system of formal study was set up, open and competitive examinations for doctors were also instituted, and for the first time the science was able to begin sifting out unqualified quacks who had been dishonouring the profession, and making a lot of money, by defrauding the sick with phoney medical advice and prescriptions.

The pharmacopoeia of herbal medicine was again updated and revised by Tang medical scholars, and the first illustrated version appeared with drawings of the various plants and herbs. The dietary link with medicine was advanced by one of the foremost physicians of the era, Dr Sun Simiao, a dedicated man who turned down the requests of the first two emperors of Tang to become their personal physician, preferring instead to concentrate on his practice and research among the diseases of the common people.

In this field, Dr Sun was able to specialise, and distinguish himself, in the treatment of sicknesses caused by malnutrition. And his study and use of diet as a medical therapy produced treatments that are among those proved accurate by Western research some 1,000 to 1,300 years after his time. For example, he prescribed seaweed and extracts of deer and lamb thyroid—all high in iodine content—as a dietary supplement for mountain folk suffering from goiter, or enlarged thyroid glands. He also cured beriberi with calf and lamb liver, almond, wild Sichuan pepper and wheat germ—treatments that are all rich in vitamins A and B.

These and other developments of Tang dynasty medicine were advanced and refined in the Song dynasty (A.D. 960-1279). New medical schools were established, their curricula expanded, and a more rigid and comprehensive system of examinations brought in. Medical students were now required to treat sick faculty members, bureaucrats and soldiers as part of their practical studies, and the results were applied to their examination scores at the end of each year. There was a general elevation of Chinese arts and science during the Song period, along with a resurgence of Confucian philosophy, especially its ethics. These twin pillars of culture and integrity raised the standards of medicine as well: respect for physicians grew, and their position in the monolithic pyramidal structure of Chinese society was now one of eminence. In fact the term *ren yi*, or "benevolent doctor," was coined by the Song dynasty's neo-Confucianists. It was also during this time that the physician and his ancient forefather, the herb-gathering mountain mystic, went their separate ways, for the Confucianists cold-shouldered the intense and austere spiritualism of the confirmed Taoists.

The Song era saw all the empire's herbal prescriptions standardised. It also saw the herbal treatments expanded to include pastes and poultices, and pills—powdered herbs bound and coated with thick honey. Technology also raced ahead under Song rule, and paper and woodblock printing presses were developed, with the result that the pharmacopoeia of herbal medicine was revised four times—the last Song edition listing almost 1,000 medicines.

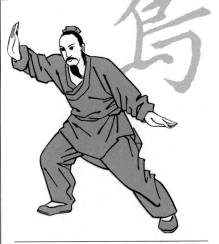

OPPOSITE Hua Tuo, the renowned Han dynasty physician, used a "narcotic" to anaesthesise General Guan Yu when he removed a arrow head from his arm. ABOVE *Tai ji* exercises depict the stance of the bear (top left), tiger (bottom left), deer (centre), monkey (top) and bird (above).

23

The Mongols of Genghis Khan conquered China in 1260 and ruled the empire from Beijing for 108 years. Medicine, along with many other fields of Chinese learning, fell into a period of dormancy under the Mongol Yuan rule, but the following Ming dynasty restored Chinese sovereignty and triggered a cultural renaissance which was to affect all areas of the intellectual world. The Ming period was one of the great adventure, marked by the celebrated voyages of trade and discovery under the eunuch admiral, Zheng He—voyages that took huge Chinese junk fleets as far as, and perhaps beyond, the Cape of Good Hope. Medical science flourished again and there emerged another giant of herbal medicine, Dr Li Shizhen (A.D. 1517-1593), who produced the classic herbal encyclopaedia, *Ben Cao Gang Mu, General Outlines and Divisions of Herbal Medicine*, that remains to this day the key reference work of the science. It took Dr Li 27 years to complete this huge book, during which he travelled all over China in search of medical herbs. The result was 52 book-scrolls listing no less than 1,892 medicines. It was not ony widely distributed throughout China but was also translated into Japanese, Korean, Vietnamese, English, French, German and Russian, and is said to have had some influence on the studies and revolutionary theories of Charles Darwin.

In this respect, Dr Li's works marked the beginning of a cultural exchange between Chinese and Western medical science. The Venetian adventurers who had followed Marco Polo's path to the "Middle Kingdom" brought Western science and technology to the Ming court and translated many European medical books into Chinese. In return, the vast pharmacopoeia of herbal medicine was thrown open to the West. During the Manchu dynasty which supplanted the Mings and drew cultural bars on the age of adventure, this exchange was intensified by British and European military adventures aimed at forcing the insular, xenophobic Manchus to open China's doors to free trade and modernisation. In 1790 a Dutch botanist went

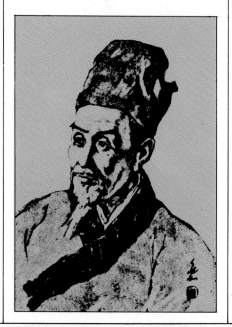

Dr Li Shizhen, the Ming dynasty medical scholar, who worked for 27 years on his classic herbal encyclopaedia.

to Japan to study oriental plants and took many back to grow and experiment with in Holland. In fact, what he took back were Chinese medical herbs which had earlier spread to Japan to form the basis of Japanese herbal medicine. And so, herbs and plants like rhubarb, hydrasts, gentian, licorice, aconite, field mint, ginger and yellow vetch—all used for centuries by the Chinese physicians—made their way into European and British pharmacology.

With Western military and missionary incursion in China, herbal medicine came under growing pressure from Western medicine. British doctors opened up practices in Guangzhou and the other trading concessions. Missionary doctors such as John Kerr of Glasgow introduced Chinese translations of Western medical journals into Guangzhou and Shanghai. After the collapse of the Manchus and the establishment of the Republic of China, Western medicine took its place alongside traditional herbal science in new Chinese medical schools set up in Shanghai and other major cities. Inevitably, the time came when Chinese and Western medicine faced each other in direct confrontation, and this struggle came to a head in 1929 when Chinese doctors who had studied Western medicine in Japan returned home to demand that traditional herbal medicine be banned. Such was the strength of tradition, however, that the demand was met with vehement opposition throughout all classes of Chinese society. A meeting of physicians from all over China was held in Shanghai, and it elected a delegation to go before the Nationalist government in Nanjing to plead the case for herbal medicine. It succeeded in winning the government's support, and to commemorate the victory, the date of that fateful petition, March 17, was declared "Chinese Doctors' Day". Four years later the government paid tribute to the importance of the science by establishing the Central Chinese Hospital in Nanjing, and a chief justice of the Supreme Court, Chiao Yi-tang was appointed president and charged with the duty of further systemising and promoting herbal medicine.

Thus, this 5,000-year-old science survived, and there now began a process of scientific review that has

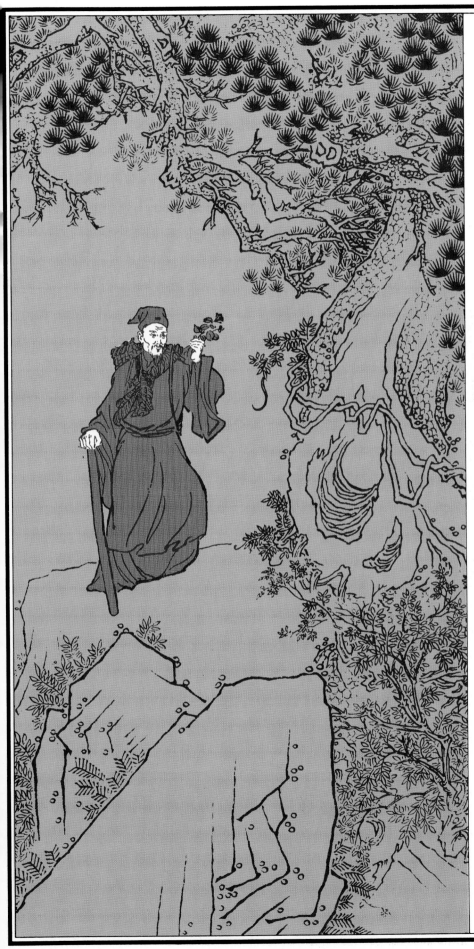

brought the theory and practice of the medicine into the laboratories of the twentieth century. The first step toward this review was taken at a conference of the League of Nations in Geneva in 1931 when a committee was set up to undertake research on Chinese medicine. At about the same time, the science was given a strong academic boost in the West by a wealthy American businessman, G.M. Gest, who had an eye disease that was healed by a Chinese physician after all other efforts had failed. Mr Gest's gratitude was such that he collected some 75,000 volumes of Chinese medical books

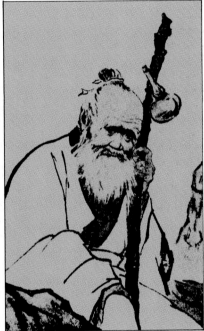

and established the Gest Oriental Library at Princeton University.

Western research has since confirmed much of the science of Chinese herbal medicine. It remains now for an historic marriage to take place between Western medical technology and both the curative powers and the undeniably humane and spiritual precepts of Chinese healing.

OPPOSITE: Dr. Li Shizhen, compiler of the classic herbal encyclopaedia. *Ben Cao Gang Mu, General Outliner and Divisions of Herbal Medicine.* LEFT Gathering and tasting "the myriad herbs." ABOVE Dr Sun Simiao, the Tang dynasty medical scholar, who first advanced the theory of a link between diet and health.

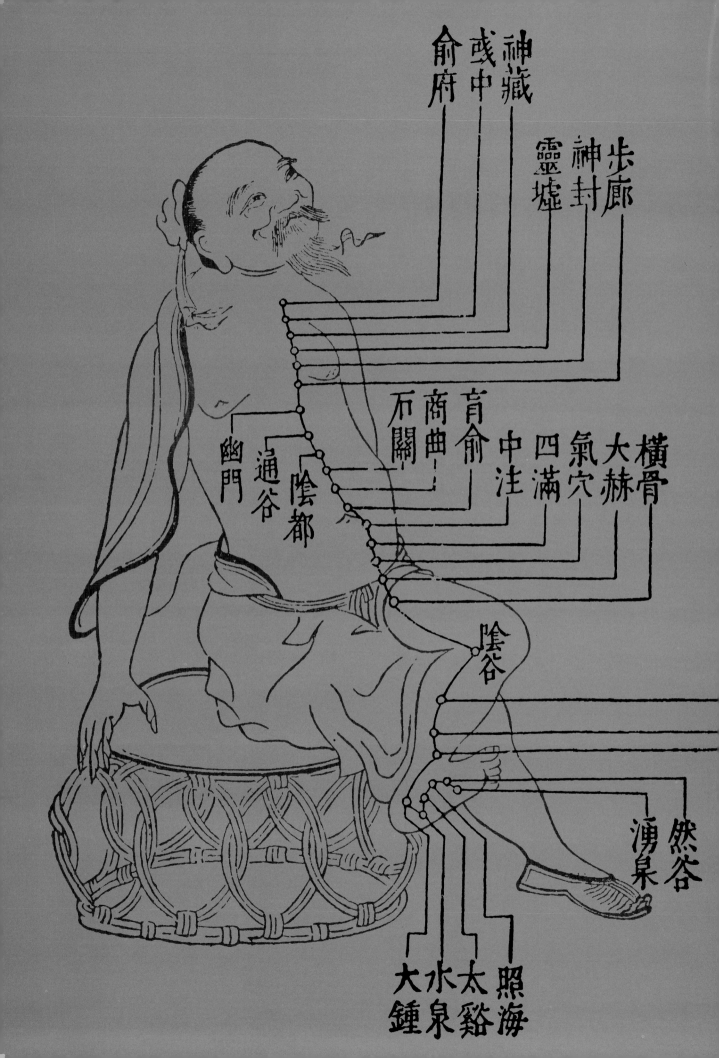

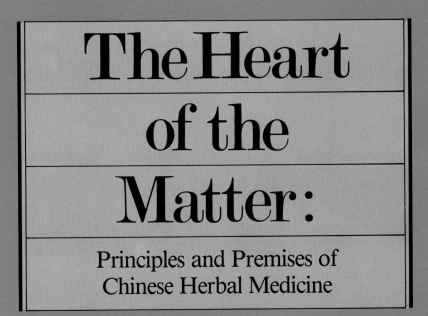

Chapter III

The Heart
of the
Matter:

Principles and Premises of
Chinese Herbal Medicine

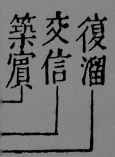

he cosmic element prevails throughout the entire field of traditional Chinese medicine. The same concepts and terminology which define the traditional Chinese view of the universe are also used to describe the myriad phenomena of health and disease. The Chinese regard the human body and all of its functions as a microcosm of the grand cosmic order. They believe that the same forces which permeate the universe and animate nature in all its variety are also at work in man. The principles and premises of Chinese medicine are drawn directly from traditional Taoist philosophy, China's most ancient and singular school of thought.

The Chinese have always learned from empirical observation. They have little faith in rigid systems drawn from abstract theories, such as those that prevail in the West. Taoist thought stresses fluctuation and mutability and explains all natural phenomena in terms of the constant ebb and flow of cosmic forces. Western minds, in contrast, prefer to deal with structured concepts, fixed quantities, and absolute laws. Consequently, the principles and premises of Chinese medicine, especially the concepts and terms used to explain them, are difficult for the average Westerner to absorb at first glance. Closer scrutiny usually reveals the soundness, sense and profundity of the insights which permeate the system. The symbolic terms used in Chinese medicine, drawn directly from nature or borrowed from Taoist philosophy, have an exotic charm and poetic tone. The symbolic nature should always be kept in mind. In the following pages Chinese medical concepts are presented as clearly and concisely as possible and woven into a comprehensive theoretical description of the inner workings of Chinese herbal medicine.

QI AND THE FOUR VITAL BODILY HUMOURS

The major premise of Chinese medical theory is that all the forms of life in the universe are animated by an essential life-force or vital energy called *qi*. *Qi* also means "breath" and "air" and is similar to the Hindu concept of *prana*. Invisible, tasteless, odourless, and formless, *qi* nevertheless permeates the entire cosmos. *Qi* is transferable and transmutable: digestion extracts *qi* from food and drink and transfers it to the body; breathing extracts *qi* from air and transfers it to the lungs. When these two forms of *qi* meet in the bloodstream, they transmute to form human-*qi*, which then circulates throughout the body as vital energy. It is the quality, quantity, and balance of your *qi* that determines your state of health and span of life.

There are many kinds of *qi*: "hot-*qi*" and "cold-*qi*;" "yin-*qi*" and "yang-*qi*;" "dry-*qi*" and "moist-*qi*;" and many others. There is the "evil-*qi*" emanating from swamps (miasma) which causes disease and the "pure-*qi*" of mountain mists which promotes health and prolongs life. The key to maintaining optimum health is a natural and harmonious balance among the vital energies within the body, as well as between those of the body and the external environment. For example, over-indulgence in peppery, highly-spiced "hot" foods generally results in a build-up of *huo qi* (fire-energy) in the body, with all the attendant symptoms of dry lips, parched mouth and throat, distended chest, and constipation. These symptoms would be far worse in mid-summer, when the

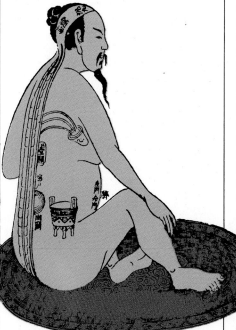

environment is dominated by heat, than in mid-winter, when the body needs extra heat-inducing foods to balance the excess cold outside. To eliminate these "hot" symptoms and restore the proper energy balance, one need only ingest a few "cool" foods such as water-melon, citrus fruits, white turnips, etc. There is a constant co-mingling of the various types of energy within and without the body. The person who is aware of this can adjust the balance of energies in his body on a daily or even hourly basis with diet, exercise, breathing, and herbal medicines.

The quantity, quality, and balance of a person's *qi* are as variable as the weather and are significantly influenced by changes in season and climate. The most important factors concerning *qi*, however, are the food and drink we consume and the air we breathe. This explains the great importance of diet and breathing exercises in the Taoist system of health and longevity. Quality and quantity of *qi* are further influenced by the condition of the organs which absorb *qi*. If the stomach and lungs are not functioning properly, they are unable to extract and absorb vital energy in pure form and sufficient quantity. The result is that the entire body suffers and energy deficiency arises. Many common ailments are simply due to insufficient levels and inferior quality of vital energy in the system. This is why astute Chinese doctors first look to their patients' general life-styles and daily habits for clues. *Qi*-deficient ailments can usually be corrected with a combination of proper diet, exercise, breathing, and hygiene. Only when a problem has become so serious that it impairs the functions of vital organs and glands, does the Chinese physician resort to curative herbal medications. Due to their natural affinities for certain parts of the body, the *qi* extracted from medicinal plants goes straight to the organ or gland for which they have been prescribed. There they act to restore the diseased organ to its orginal tissue tone and natural functions, in the process redressing the attendant imbalances of vital energy.

The original and ideal state of one's collective vital energies is called *yuan qi*, literally "primordial vital energy." From the day we are born until our last day of life, a gradual but inexorable process of deterioration and dissipation of our *yuan qi* takes place. The rate of this process determines our life-span. The Taoists, in seeking longevity, developed techniques to slow down the dissipation of their primordial vital energy and redress the constant deterioration of organs and glands. In short, they sought to slow down the aging process. Breathing and kung-fu exercises, diet and herbal medicine all work to increase the quantity and improve the quality of one's vital energy and to repair damage to vital

and moistens the skin, controls the opening and closing of pores and protects the body from invasion by "outside evil-*qi*." When internal nourishing-*qi* is deficient, the body is susceptible to weaknesses or diseases (or both) of the vital organs. When the surface protecting-*qi* is too weak, the body becomes vulnerable to outside invasion by wind, cold, damp, and other environmental "excesses" which can cause disease.

Qi is one of the four bodily humours and by far the most important one. The others are blood *xue*, vital essence *jing*, and fluid *jin ye*. Blood is formed together with

ach and small intestine. It constitutes the creative force inside the body and takes two forms: life-essence and semen-essence. Life-essence is stored in the kidneys, which secrete it into the bloodstream as needed. It controls growth, development, decay and death. In terms of Western medical science, "kidneys" here mean the vital glands which straddle the kidneys—the renal and suprarenal glands. "Life-essence" refers to the vital hormones secreted from these glands, which control many vital life functions.

Semen-essence refers to the spermatozoa in males and the ova in females. Embryos formed from the union of male and female semen-essence are nourished by the life-essence also formed by this union. After birth, the child produces its own life-essence by digestion. According to traditional Chinese views, the sexual-*jing* in girls matures at two times seven years, around age fourteen, and deteriorates at seven times seven, around age forty-nine. Likewise, the *jing* of boys matures at two times eight years, age sixteen, and begins to lose potency at eight times eight, age sixty-four. The life and semen types of vital essence are closely related, are both stored in and around the kidneys, and manifest themselves as general as well as sexual vitality.

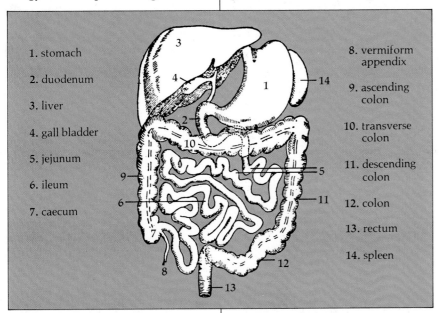

1. stomach
2. duodenum
3. liver
4. gall bladder
5. jejunum
6. ileum
7. caecum

8. vermiform appendix
9. ascending colon
10. transverse colon
11. descending colon
12. colon
13. rectum
14. spleen

organs caused by disease, weakness, or natural deterioration. This process is called *bu yuan qi*, or "tonifying the primordial vital energies," a cardinal principle and primary purpose of Chinese herbal medicine.

After *qi* has been converted to human-*qi* in the body, it takes the two forms of nourishing-*qi*, *ying qi* and protecting-*qi*, *wei qi*. "Nourishing-*qi* is produced from the purest parts of the food and drink we digest, and circulates throughout the body with the blood. It nourishes organs, glands, nerves, bones, and other tissues. Protecting-*qi* is complementary to nourishing-*qi*. It is produced from the coarser products of digestion and cannot penetrate the delicate walls of the blood vessels. Instead, it circulates around the surface of the body in the subcutaneous tissues just below the skin. It warms

nourishing-*qi* from the most refined products of digestion, and they travel together in the circulatory system to nourish the body. The movement of blood is controlled by *qi*: "*Qi* is the general of the blood; if *qi* moves, then the blood moves," according to the ancient texts. *Qi* can be regulated with breathing exercises. You'll notice that if you take a slow, deep breath, sink it down to your abdomen, and hold it a few seconds, your pulse-rate will slow down considerably. As you slowly, evenly release the breath, circulation accelerates, expanding until the pulse can be felt throbbing to the extremities and up to the brain. The importance of proper breathing is largely due to *qi*'s control over blood circulation.

Vital-essence *jing* is also produced by the transforming effects of *qi* on digested food and drink in the stom-

The other vital bodily humour is a fluid, *jin ye*, which is also extracted from digested food and drink. After being acted upon by *qi*, it acquires the special quality of life which distinguishes bodily fluid from ordinary water and liquids. The amount and balance of fluid in the body is a vital health factor. Too much or too little will upset the natural equilibrium of yin and yang, and it is therefore constantly regulated by the organs. The small intestine separates pure from impure fluids, the kidneys control the amount to be used or rejected, and the bladder stores and expels waste and excess fluid. Various organs convert fluid to different forms for different uses. The liver, which is associated with eye functions converts fluid to tears. The

OPPOSITE Early illustration of the "Stream of Life," the main bodily functions. ABOVE The internal organs.

spleen, which has digestive functions, produces saliva from fluid. The lungs form mucus. The heart transforms fluid to sweat and the kidneys convert fluid to urine.

The Chinese distinguish two types of bodily fluid: clear-fluid *jin* and thick-fluid *ye*. Clear-fluid circulates with protecting-*qi*, moistening the flesh and skin and appearing as normal, clear perspiration on the surface. Thick-fluid travels with nourishing-*qi* and blood lubricating the sinews and joints and filling the marrow of bones and the hollows of the brain. It appears on the body's surface as the greasy excretion of sweat glands.

Qi, blood, vital-essence, and fluid are all closely associated. A deficiency in one inevitably has adverse effects on the others. Nevertheless, *qi*—the great energiser of the body—remains most vital. It is the action of *qi* on digested food and drink which actually produces blood, vital-essence, and fluid, and *qi* moves together with these substances through the body. In addition, *qi* is the only one of the four vital substances which can be obtained other than by digestion of food and drink: it is also extracted from air by the lungs. One reason that proper diet has always been so important in Chinese medicine is that the quality and quantity of the other three substances depend entirely upon food and drink.

YIN AND YANG

Yin and yang are familiar Chinese terms to Western ears. The concepts these terms embody are central to Taoist philosophy as well as to Chinese medicine. The theory of yin and yang pervades every aspect of Chinese life and thought. The balance between these two primordial cosmic forces is viewed as the key factor in all natural phenomena and life processes.

The interplay between yin and yang sparks all change and movement in the universe. Yin represents the negative, passive force. It is female in nature, dark, low-lying, contractive, descending, and is symbolised by water. Yang symbolises the positive, active force. It is male in nature, bright, high-flying, expan-

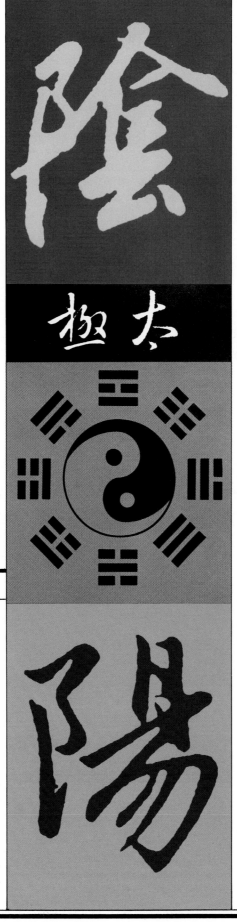

sive, ascending, and is represented by fire. Of the two forces, Taoists believe yin to be superior and stronger. Citing the analogy of fire and water, they point out that fire tends to flare up quickly, giving a brief appearance of great power, but is easily extinguished by water. Water, on the other hand, is indestructible, fills everything, and eventually wears down even the hardest rock. Water can be gradually warmed and even aroused to the boiling point by fire—if fire doesn't burn itself out first. It has the power to absorb and retain yang energy for a long time. Ever since the term first appeared over 3,000 years ago, yin has been placed before yang in word order.

Yin and yang are mutually dependent forces: one cannot exist without the other. The ideal state of nature, including health, is a harmonious balance between the two. When yang is in excess, yin tends to recede. When yin overflows, yang tends to retreat. The net total, however, is always the same.

Yin and yang transmute into their own opposites when they reach critical levels of excess. This concept is best illustrated by the classical Chinese symbol for the cosmic balance of yin and yang. The dark yin and bright yang are depicted in perfect balance. Note that where yin tapers off and becomes weak, yang is at its strongest, and where yang tapers off, yin builds up. Both yin and yang contain the germ of their own opposite within themselves, as symbolised by the white and black dots. It is the seed of yin within the yang and the seed of yang within the yin that gives impetus to their constant flux and the ceaseless waxing and waning of the two forces.

The key to understanding the theory of yin and yang is the concept of relative balance. The Chinese do not believe in absolutes or ideals: everything is relative, flexible, and changing. What may be a perfect yin-yang balance in the body during summer, for example, would be inappropriate during winter, when cold yin-forces dominate the environment and the body requires extra warming yang-energy. When the body fills with excess yang-energy, driving out the yin to the point of deficiency, then cooling yin medicines and foods are prescribed to restore the relative balance. Similarly, if yin rises and yang recedes, warming yang medications are required to re-establish the proper relative balance. Within certain limits, the body adjusts the relative balance of yin-yang automatically. When imbalances reach critical levels, medication is required. For optimum health it is best to avoid yin-yang imbalances with basic preventive care such as proper diet and exercise combined with careful attention to changes in season, weather, and geography.

Yin and yang each have their own domains within the human body, although these spheres of influence intersect. Yin controls the internal, the lower, and the front portions of the body, while yang dominates the external, upper, and back parts. Half the vital organs belong to yin and half to yang. Yin governs blood, yang governs energy-qi. Yin descends, while yang ascends. Innate instincts are yin, and learned skills belong to yang. However, these distinctions always remain relative, never absolute. For example, it is said that the body's exterior is yang and its interior yin; yet at the same time the exterior surface of each internal organ is governed by yang, while its interior is ruled by yin. Man is yang and woman is yin, but both man and woman have elements of both. Yin-yang is simply a symbolic way of designating opposite forces that are at work in everything from the solar system down to the minutest cell of the body. The relative balance between these cosmic forces within the body and between the body and the environment is the most basic regulator of health and longevity.

Foods and herbal medicines redress yin-yang imbalances by supplementing the deficient element. One example of basic preventive care based on the yin-yang theory is to adjust the diet according to the season: in summer, cooling yin foods should be increased in the diet and overly hot yang foods avoided. In winter, plenty of warming yang foods should be included in the diet, and in extreme cold a few warming yang herbal medications should be consumed regularly as well. Since each item in the *ben cao* has its own

relatively yin or yang nature, every item in an herbal prescription affects the body's yin-yang balance to some degree. Chinese physicians engage nature in an extraordinary balancing act. After determining the cause and nature of a patient's energy imbalances, they must weigh such general factors as weather, season, and geography with the factors that are unique to the patient's condition, balancing the whole act with appropriate herbal prescriptions and dietary advice.

THE FIVE ELEMENTS

Since ancient times, the Chinese have divided the world into five symbolic elements: Wood, Fire, Earth, Metal, and Water. Everything on earth is dominated by one of these elements, and their constant interplay, comined with those of yin and yang, explain all change and activity in nature. *The Internal Book of Huang Di*, China's oldest medical treatise, states: "The five elements Wood, Fire, Earth, Metal, and Water encompass all the phenomena of nature. It is a symbolism that applies itself equally to man." Note the word "symbolism."

The primeval forces represented by the Five Elements interact in set patterns according to their natural relationships. Each force has a generative and a subjugative influence on one other force and, in turn, is generated or subjugated by a different one. While these relationships are symbolic, it is perhaps easiest to understand them in literal terms. The generative cycle proceeds as follows: Wood burns to generate Fire; Fire produces ashes, which generates Earth; Earth generates Metal, which can be mined from the ground; when heated, Metal becomes molten, like Water; and Water promotes growth of plants, thereby generating Wood.

The negative, subjugative cycle is complementary to the positive, generative one. Plants, represented by Wood, subjugate Earth by breaking up the soil and depleting its nutrients; Earth subjugates Water by containing it in one place and soiling its clarity; Water subjugates Fire by extinguishing it; Fire subjugates Metal by melting it; and Metal subjugates Wood by cutting it.

Based on the generative-subjugative cycles, the Five Elements interact to form complex relationships, the most important of which are the "mother-son" and the "victor-vanquished" relationships. Mother-son connections are based on the generative cycle: Fire is mother to son Earth, which it generates, but Fire is son to mother Wood, which generates it; Wood is mother to son Fire, but Wood is son to mother Water; etc. The subjugative cycle determines the victor-vanquished relationship: Fire is vanquished by Water but is victor over Wood; Wood is vanquished by Metal but is victor over

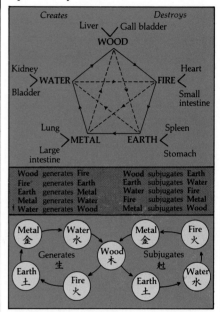

Earth, and so forth. It must always be remembered that the Five Elements, as well as other traditional Chinese descriptions of the world, are symbolic representations of fundamental natural forces. The most important aspect of these forces is their interplay.

Each vital organ belongs by nature to one of the Five Elements. Thus, the fundamental relations among the Five Elements are the key to understanding how the vital organs interact and influence each other. The generative-subjugative cycle also explains how external environmental factors affect each organ and the body as a whole. Using herbal medicines, Chinese

OPPOSITE The characters for yin (top) and yang (bottom), with the *Tai ji*, the symbol for the balance of the two forces, in between. ABOVE The traditional Five Elements and their relationship to health.

31

doctors manipulate these natural relationships to adjust energy imbalances caused by excess or deficiency of these forces in the body.

Chinese medical views regarding the vital internal organs are based on the theories of yin and yang and the Five Elements and do not correspond exactly to Western anatomical science. Cutting open a human body, dead or alive, was considered a grave insult to the person's ancestors. Therefore, dissecting corpses and performing internal surgery were generally taboo in China up to the twentieth century. Instead, Chinese physicians observed external manifestations of internal

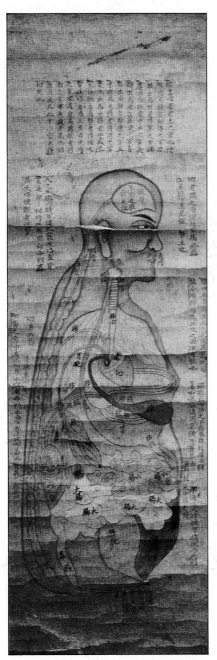

activities to gradually determine how the vital organs interact. The locations of the organs were established by common sense, comparisons to animals, and their connections to external, visible parts of the body.

Though not as physically detailed as Western anatomy, the Chinese frame of reference is remarkably precise in tracing the sources and courses of disease in the body. Since internal surgery was unheard of, the exact anatomical location of every organ, gland, vein, and artery was not important. What was important were the exact functional relationships among the organs, glands, and other parts of the body, and these have been firmly established by Chinese medical practice. Time and again the basic natural relationships of yin and yang and the Five Elements prove to be reliable guides in both diagnosis and treatment of disease.

Yin-yang and the Five Elements tie Chinese medicine directly to traditional Chinese philosophy and describe the human body in terms of the universal patterns of nature. This syncretic, symbiotic, symbolic approach to health and disease is a unique, profound feature of traditional Chinese medicine.

THE VITAL ORGANS

The functioning relationships among the vital organs are key factors in the Chinese approach to the diagnosis and treatment of disease. Their predictable interactions, based on yin-yang and the Five Elements, permit the experienced Chinese doctor to

diagnose the causes of disease and weakness, and to effect cures by evaluating the patterned connections and prescribing herbal medicines.

The Chinese refer to the vital organs as the *wu zang* and *liu fu* (the five "solid" and six "hollow" organs). With the exception of *san jiao*—the "three-points" or "triple-warmer"—the organs correspond to those of Western anatomy. The triple-warmer, one of the six hollow organs, consists of the openings to the stomach, small intestine, and bladder. As such, it is not, strictly speaking, an independent organ in the Western sense, but rather an energy system which deals with the passing of food and fluid. Later, a sixth solid organ was added to correspond to the triple-warmer and balance the system. This is the pericardium, the sack which surrounds the heart. Because the triple-warmer and the pericardium are not vital organs in the traditional Western sense, and since they are used primarily in acupuncture rather than herbal therapy, we will limit our discussion to the familiar ten: heart, lungs, liver, kidney, spleen (the five "solid" or yin organs); small intestine, large intestine, gall-bladder, bladder, stomach (the five "hollow" or yang organs).

These ten organs are divided into five coupled pairs. Each pair consists of a solid yin organ and a corresponding hollow yang organ, and each pair is dominated by one of the Five Elements. All other parts of the body reflect the condition and activities of the vital organs. According to the Five Elements, each of the five coupled pairs is identified with other parts of the body and with other basic natural factors which reflect or influence their activities. These factors are outlined in the chart opposite. Note that a fifth season, "mid-summer," is included to correspond to the element Earth and its attendant phenomena. The Chinese love balance and are suspicious of anything that is lop-sided.

While there may be some doubt as to the accuracy of a few of the factors in this chart, there is no doubt that most of them are correct and represent real relationships in nature. This chart is used successfully by Chinese doctors in both diagnosis and treatment.

Take, for example, the liver, which belongs to the element Wood. Western medicine agrees that persons suffering from liver ailments often have symptons of foggy vision with black spots, muscular spasms, and blemished nails. On the Chinese chart sight, muscles, and nails all belong to Wood and reflect liver functions. The emotions associated with Wood are anger and depression. Persons with volatile, over-active livers are prone to violent fits of anger followed by bouts of depression and they often shout (Wood sound) at others.

The factors associated with each of the Five Elements invariably reflect the activity of the related organs and, in turn, can be used to influence them. A child who suffers from chronic fear (Water emotion) tends to wet his bed (urine belongs to Water), and therefore he probably has weak kidneys (Water organ). Trying to cure his fear and his bedwetting with comforting words, stern warnings, or other psychological means, will prove frustrating, perhaps even futile, for both parent and child—if indeed the problem lies in weak kidneys. Tonifying the kidneys with herbs, or herbs and acupuncture, should quickly eliminate the symptoms of fear and incontinence. Chinese medicine is still well ahead of Western medicine in tracing and treating the physical causes of mental disturbances.

The possibilities for using these patterned relationships are endless.

OPPOSITE Internal organs as depicted on an ancient anatomical chart. (*By courtesy of the Wellcome Trustees*). ABOVE a block-print showing acupuncture points for liver treatment.

For example, a person who suffers from chronic depression (Wood emotion) can often be cured simply by treating his liver, for depression is a clear manifestation of liver dysfunction. A person with a very red complexion (Fire colour) who laughs a lot (Fire sound) probably has an over-fired heart (Fire organ). In such a case, the heart should be sedated with appropriate herbs. However, another way to treat this case is to use the victor-vanquished relationship of Water to Fire by tonifying the kidneys (Water organ). Since Water vanquishes Fire, the heart will be sedated by the tonified kidneys. Because there are so many related factors and possibilities, Chinese doctors must have a detailed account of each patient's dietary, physical, and emotional habits. Only broad clinical experience, combined with a thorough grasp of the principles involved, enables the physician to weigh the many relevant factors for accurate diagnosis and treatment.

The yin organs, which "store but do not transmit," are considered more

vital than the Yang organs, "which transform but do not retain." Coupled organs are connected to one another by meridians, or energy channels, along which their vital energies flow. The meridians of coupled organs meet in the fingers, toes, and head. The yin-yang coupling of organs is not arbitrary. It is based on their actual functional relationships, as established by observation over many centuries.

Before going on to discuss how the connections among the organs are used in Chinese medical diagnosis and treatment, a brief description of the organs themselves is in order. Following the Chinese mode, the five yin organs (which house the five attributes of spirit, human-soul, animal-soul, mind, and will-power)

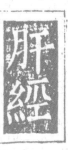

are described according to their vital functions, while their five yang counterparts are given secondary importance:

HEART: Called the "Chief of the Vital Organs", the heart regulates the other organs by controlling circulation of blood. It houses the spirit and thus governs one's moods and clarity of thought. It is closely connected to liver functions by the generative mother-son relationship of Wood to Fire. Heart activity is reflected on the colour of the face and tongue: a dark, reddish colour indicates excess heart-energy while a pale, grey colour reflects deficient heart-energy. The heart is coupled with the small intestine, which separates the pure from the impure products of digestion, controls the ratio of liquid to solid wastes, and absorbs nutrients from digested food and drink.

LIVER: The liver stores blood and regulates the amount to be circulated by the heart. When man moves, the blood travels to several meridians; when man is still, the blood returns to the liver. During sleep, blood is enriched with energy in the liver and distributed to the rest of the body during activity. The liver houses the human soul, which is said to enter the foetus at the moment of birth. The popular Chinese term of endearment *xin gan* (literally "heart-liver"), which means "dear" or "sweetheart," is derived from the fact that these two organs house the most precious of human attributes: spirit and human soul. The liver is the centre of metabolism, life's most vital function, and therefore its condition is perhaps most responsible for our overall sense of physical and mental well-being. While liver dysfunction causes symptoms of anger and depression, a healthy liver is also particularly sensitive to psychosomatic injury caused by prolonged emotional fits of anger or depression. Liver condition is reflected in the eyes, muscles, finger- and toe-nails. It is coupled with the gall-bladder, whose functions are closely related to, and often inseparable from, those of the liver. The gall-bladder is called the "true and upright official who excels in making decisions." Planning and deciding are said to be governed by combined liver and gall-bladder activity.

SPLEEN: The spleen controls the "moving and transforming" of pure vital essence extracted by the stomach from food and drink. It is responsible for distributing nutrients and *qi* to the rest of the body. Spleen dysfunction is indicated by weakness or emaciation of the skin, flesh, and limbs. The spleen houses the mind. It is coupled with the stomach, which is described as "the sea of water and nourishment and the controller of rotting and ripening of liquid and solid food." If the spleen fails to move

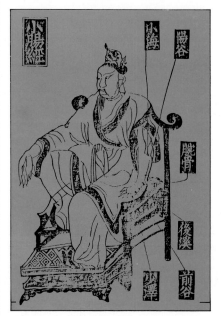

and transform, the stomach will back up and fail to digest properly. If the stomach fails to rot and ripen food and water, the spleen cannot move and transform nutrition and *qi*. The harmonious functioning of these two organs is vital for proper digestion and distribution of nutrition. Western medical science does not assign the spleen any digestive functions and recognises no functional connection to the stomach. It has been suggested therefore that the digestive functions assigned to the spleen in the Chinese system may in fact include those of the pancreas, which is located nearby and secretes such vital digestive juices as trypsin, maltase, lapase, and others.

LUNGS: The lungs control vital energy, *qi*, in both senses of the word, namely energy and breath. The lungs govern breathing, and when breath is insufficient, so is energy. The lungs extract *qi* from the air and transfer it to the blood through the alveoli. "Man's breathing combines the pure vital essence of Heaven (air) and Earth (food and water) in order to form the true human-*qi* of the body." The lungs house the animal-soul, which is said to enter the embryo at the moment of conception. The condition of the lungs is closely associated with that of the skin, a fact well known to Western medicine. In many animals, skin performs important respiratory functions. Lung dysfunctions usually manifest themselves as skin problems. The lungs are coupled with the large intestine, which "controls the transmitting and drainage of the dregs." Pneumonia and influenza are generally accompanied by constipation, while the latter ailment usually causes distension of the chest.

KIDNEYS: The kidneys control water, receive the vital essence of the *wu zang* and *liu fu*—vital organs—and store it. The kidneys store both life-essence and semen-essence. Excess liquid sent by the small intestine is converted by the kidneys to urine and passed on to its coupled organ, the bladder, for storage and expulsion. Growth and development of bones and marrow are connected to the kidneys. Since the brain is the "meeting point for all marrow," the kidneys influence brain function. They house the attribute of will-power. When kidney-*qi* is deficient, the symptoms are amnesia, insomnia, mental confusion, and a constant ringing inside the ears. Kidneys control the loins, lumbar region, and sacral areas of the body, and their dysfunction often causes lower back pains and the inability to straighten up. The kidneys are closely related to the adrenal cortex which produces the cortisone hormones as well as sex hormones like androgen, oestrogen, and progesterone. Therefore, the kidneys and surrounding glands control all sexual functions. A recent study in America has revealed that frequent sexual intercourse helps relieve the pain of rheumatism in elderly people by stimulating production of cortisone through sexual excitation of the adrenal cortex. The therapeutic applications of sexual intercourse have long been known in China. The kidneys and bladder function closely together in moving, converting, storing, and expelling excess fluids from the system.

The above is a simplified account of the vital organs according to traditional Chinese medical theory. A full accounting would require a book in itself but it can be seen from this brief sketch that the Chinese lay emphasis on the functions of the vital organs, and the functional relationships among them. Western medicine, in contrast, stresses the location, structure, and physical description of the organs. What concerns the Chinese physician is the elaborate interplay of basic forces which ultimately regulate all bodily functions, not microscopic anatomy, biochemical formulas, or isolated phenomena. While Western medical science has managed to analyse and isolate every single functional structure in the body, right down to individual cells, nuclei, and beyond, it has less ideas of what makes the whole system tick and function harmoniously. Chinese medicine has dwelled on such questions as what is the nature of the vital energy at the root of all life? how does it work? what factors influence it? what forms does it take? Both physical and mental symptoms of health and disease are viewed as concrete manifestations of potent natural forces and vital energies at work inside the body. In treating disease, the Chinese believe they must exert a balancing on these forces and energies, rather than simply eliminate the symptoms of the disease.

Unfortunately, Western science does not readily accept as real things that cannot be directly detected and measured with the senses, or with equipment to aid them. Chinese doctors are quick to point out, however, that even the senses are mere physical entities controlled by the same unseen vital energy as the rest of the body. At best, the sense can be used to detect physical manifestations of cosmic forces and vital energy. The nature of the forces themselves has to be intuited and inferred from the evidence. The main concern of Chinese medicine during its long history has been to establish the patterns by which these forces and energies interact. To develop natural herbal techniques favourably influencing their relative balance in the body has been part of that concern.

THE VITAL CONNECTIONS

Since the Chinese emphasise the functional relationships rather than the physical anatomy of the vital organs, the means by which they influence each other is of prime importance. That the circulatory, lymphatic, and nervous systems carry blood, fluids, and messages through the body is agreed upon by both Chinese and Western medicine. However, the Chinese distinguish an additional connecting system called *jing luo* or meridians. Of all the connectors in the body, the Chinese view the meridians as the most important because they circulate and transmit the body's most vital substance—*qi*, the essential energy of life.

There has been much speculation in Western medical circles regarding the mechanics of the meridian complex. The most common Western view is that meridians are actually fibres of the autonomous nervous system, and that *qi* is actually the electrical phenomenon aroused by the stimulation of the nervous system. The Chinese deny this, pointing out that *qi* also travels where there are no nerve fibres and that meridians, like *qi* itself, only manifest themselves functionally, not physically. Meridians can also be felt when vital points along them are stimulated with acupuncture. In this presentation we take the Chinese view.

There are a total of fifty-nine meridians in the body, of which twelve —the "main" meridians—dominate the others. Each of the main meridians represents a biological energy system centred around one of the twelve vital organs, including the triple-warmer and pericardium. *Qi* flows from one meridian to another in a certain order until the entire network is covered, delivering vital energy to every part of the body. Adepts of Taoist breathing techniques are able to sense and direct the flow of *qi* along the meridian complex.

Coupled yin-yang organs are directly connected by the main meridians which meet in the fingers, toes, and head. In addition, there are eight "extra", twelve "muscle" and fifteen "connecting" meridians. All are branches of the twelve main meridians and serve to distribute *qi* to those areas not covered by them. The entire complex forms a fine, intricate grid. Stimulating one of the main meridians with acupuncture or herbs has a specific effect on the connected organ as well as a general effect on the entire system. As can be seen from the below figure, there are countless combinations of connections by which organs and the

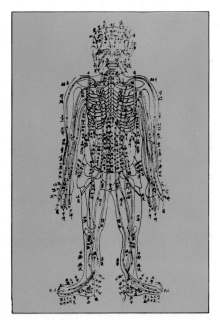

energy systems they represent can influence one another. The task of the clinical physician is to determine the most likely and most frequent patterns of interplay among the vital energies which emanate from the organs.

Chinese herbal medicine imparts its healing benefits to the body as much through the meridian complex as through the bloodstream. When an herbal prescription is ingested, its vital essence is extracted by the stomach and distributed to the blood by the spleen. After mixing with air-*qi* in the lungs to form usable human-*qi*, the herbal essence travels to the organ for which it has a natu-

OPPOSITE Block print shows acupuncture points for small intestine treatment. ABOVE Anatomical chart of acupuncture points and the course of "travelling vessels."

ral affinity and for which it has therefore been prescribed. There it has a direct biochemical effect on the organ, in turn affecting the quality and quantity of vital energy flowing along the organ's meridian. Through the meridian complex, the energy emanating from the treated organ influences other organs and parts of the body. An herbal liver tonic, for example, will improve the biochemical functions of a weak or diseased liver, tone up its damaged tissues and fortify the blood which the liver nourishes. By correcting the liver's dysfunction, the herbal tonic also corrects the imbalance of energies in the liver and tonifies liver-*qi*. Tonified liver-*qi* benefits the gall bladder through the yin-yang connection, stimulates the heart through the mother-son relationship of Wood to Fire, improves vision, muscle tone and other Wood attributes, and promotes general vitality through the minor meridian connections.

Important as the direct, immediate biochemical effects of herbal drugs are, the indirect, long-term benefits which they impart to the organ-based energy system are even more significant for health and longevity. While Western medical science acknowledges the biochemical therapeutic effects of some of the crude, knarled, ungainly items of the Chinese pharmacopoeia, it still has trouble dealing with such concepts as *qi*, pure vital essence, meridians, cosmic forces and other factors which cannot be physically dissected and measured.

The foregoing is a basic outline of the highly complex subject of meridian networks. In addition to the circulatory, lymphatic, and nervous systems, meridians form the primary communications system among the vital organs. For a very readable and comprehensive study of meridians and acupuncture, the reader is referred to Dr. Felix Mann's excellent series of books on the subject, listed in the Bibliography. Below, we will illustrate how these vital connections work with three concrete examples, dealing only with the more important yin organs.

One of the most important connections is between the heart and kidneys. They influence each other through the victor-vanquished re-

lationship of Water to Fire. It is common knowledge in Western medical pathology that heart failure is generally accompanied by renal complications, and that kidney problems usually induce heart palpitations and other Fire symptoms. If, for example, the kidneys are empty of yin-energy, they become weak and thus Water loses its subjugative control over Fire. Heart-fire flares up, inducing symptoms of restlessness, insomnia, talkativeness, and excess laughter. In this case, the kidneys should be tonified to strengthen their yin-energy, which in turn will quell the fire in the heart and restore the proper Fire-Water equilibrium.

The liver and heart interact through the mother-son relationship of Wood to Fire. The heart controls circulation of blood while the liver regulates its quality and quantity through metabolism. If the heart-*qi* is weak, the heart cannot provide sufficient circulatory power to handle the enriched blood sent up by the liver, and liver function is thus impaired. In the more colourful Chinese terminology, the Fire of the heart is insufficient to burn the Wood provided by the liver; thus, Wood piles up unburned and liver-*qi* accumulates in excess. Dizziness, spasms, pains in the joints, and anger are common symptoms of such liver-*qi* excess. The Wood-Fire equilibrium may be restored by tonifying the heart.

The interplay of energies between two organs can also occur through a third intermediary organ. The lungs and liver, for example, interact through the victory-vanquished relationship of Metal to Wood. Normally, Metal subjugates Wood, and thereby the lungs keep the liver in check. If lung-*qi* becomes deficient, Metal loses control over Wood, and the liver becomes inflamed with excess *qi*. Excess liver-*qi* (Wood) feeds the Fire of the heart through the mother-son relationship of Wood to Fire. When heart-*qi* (Fire) is in excess, it damages the lungs (Metal) through the victory-vanquished relationship of Fire to Metal. Thus, the lung (Metal), which normally subjugate the liver (Wood), can also be subjugated and damaged by the liver through the intermediary of the heart

(Fire). This case should be treated by tonifying the lungs to control the liver, sedating the liver to cool down the heart, sedating the heart to take the heat off the lungs, or some combination of these.

According to the Chinese, "everything under heaven" is animated and influenced by the same universal cosmic forces. The human body is viewed as a living microcosm of the divine pattern. Just as too much water in the atmosphere causes rain, too much water in the body causes sweating and urination. Too much heat parches and cracks the earth, just as too much heat in the body parches the throat and cracks the lips. Health and vitality depend upon the harmonious balance among these forces, and all disease begins with or causes some sort of energy imbalance. Lasting, effective cures can only be achieved by sedating excess, tonifying deficiency, cooling excess heat, warming excess cold, and otherwise redressing energy imbalance to restore the original condition of our primordial energies. This is the meaning of *bu yuan qi*.

THE CAUSES OF DISEASE

Modern Western medical science attempts to isolate purely physical factors as the cause of all diseases. Germs and bugs, bacteria and viruses, chemical compounds, and other tangible factors are blamed for virtually every illness. The Chinese, however, view many of these "causes" merely as symptoms of the disease; because a certain organ is already weak and unable to resist outside invasion, it therefore is prone to attack by germs. Killing the germs eliminates the immediate symptoms but does nothing to restore the *yuan qi* of the diseased organ and tissues. It is only a matter of time before it is attacked again.

Of course, ancient China did not have the technological means to observe and identify minute germs. But even modern practitioners of the ancient art consider the presence of germs to be a more a manifestation rather than a cause of disease. Why do germs attack some people and not others? Why do common bacterial infections invade the lungs of one patient, the knees of another, and the bowels of a third? The reason, according to Chinese theory, is that germs gather and thrive only in weakened parts of the body of patients with low resistance. Thus, the true cause of disease are those conditions which lower a patient's resistance, weaken certain parts of his body, and expose him to attack by germs. Similarly, the true cure for disease is not simply to kill germs. It is to counteract those conditions which permit disease to develop in the first place; to re-establish the body's optimum relative balance of energies and tonify the primordial energies of the weakened organs. Germs simply cannot attack strong healthy organs.

Chinese medicine attributes the cause of most diseases to external cosmological and internal emotional factors. These factors conform with and act according to the principles of yin-yang and the Five Elements. The small percentage of diseases which do not fall into either of these two categories are listed under "miscellaneous causes" such as traumatic injury, food poisoning, major epidemics, and so forth.

The external cosmological causes of disease are called the "Six Excesses" and are governed by the meteorological conditions of season and climate. "The Six Excesses are the mother of germs," states a modern treatise called *The Art of Acupuncture* by Cheng Mingchi. When certain meteorological conditions are in excess, they tend to have adverse effects on the body. Heat, damp, cold, dryness, and various combinations thereof accumulate in weakened parts of the body of patients with low resistance. It is a well known fact that each type of germ thrives only under certain exact conditions of temperature, humidity and other elements. The delicate art of fermenting wines, for example, attests to this fact. Careful control of heat, moisture, air-circulation, and other meteorological conditions regulates the activities of the yeast germs. The same is true in the body. When meteorological excesses invade a weak body, they establish the conditions favourable to the growth of germs. While Western doctors treat what they can see with their micro-

scopes, i.e., germs, Chinese doctors treat the conditions which attract and support germs. When those conditions are corrected, the germs can no longer thrive, and the disease disappears.

The Six Excesses are wind, cold, summer-heat, dampness, dryness, and fire. They are briefly described below:

WIND: Wind belongs to the element Wood and dominates in spring. In spring, the body is unaccustomed to the warm temperatures and the pores dilate easily, making it easier for "evil-wind" excess to enter the body. Symptoms of "wind-injury" are

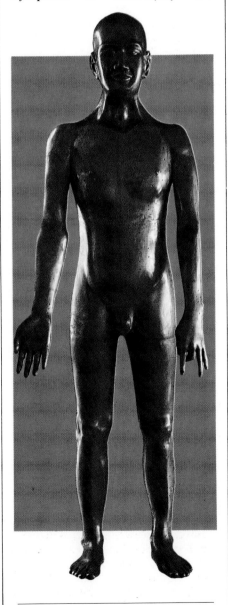

A bronze model of acupuncture points, used for training. (courtesy The Chinese University of Hongkong).

coughing, stuffy or runny nose, headache, dizziness, and sneezing. Wind often combines with heat, "wind-heat,' or cold, "wind-cold," depending on the weather, and such winds induce symptoms of both excesses. There is also an "inner-wind," unrelated to weather, which originates in the heart, liver, or kidneys due to energy imbalances. Symptoms of "inner-wind injury" are fainting, weakness, nervous spasms, blurry vision, and stiffness in the muscles and joints.

COLD: Cold is associated with the element Water and dominates in winter. Belonging to Water, cold is a "yin-evil,"which usually injures the body's yang-energy. If cold enters the exterior surface of the body, it produces symptoms of fever, aversion to cold, headache, and body pains. If it reaches the meridians, it produces muscle cramps and pains in the bones and joints. If it enters as far as the internal organs, cold-excess causes diarrhoea, vomiting, abdominal pains, and intestinal noises. "Inner-cold," again unrelated to weather, is usually caused by deficiency of yang-energy in the stomach and spleen, inducing the internal cold symptoms of nausea, diarrhoea, coldess in the limbs and a pallid complexion. Excessive consumption of cold foods ("cold" in sense of energy, not temperature) can also induce inner-cold.

SUMMER-HEAT: Summer-heat belongs to the element Fire and is predominant during the mid-summer season. Major symptoms of summer heat are excess body heat, profuse sweating, parched mouth and throat, constipation, and heart palpitations. When summer-heat combines with dampness, it produces abdominal pains, vomiting, and intestinal spasms. Iced drinks taken in the heat of mid-summer sometimes cause "yin-summer-heat." The two excesses combine in the stomach and induce symptoms of unpleasant chills, dull headache, abdominal pains, and profuse perspiration.

DAMPNESS: Dampness is associated with the element Earth and is most active in late-summer. Ailments of damp-excess can be induced by sudden exposure to fog or mists, immersion in water or exposure to rain, and living in excessively damp locations or climates. The symptoms —lethargy, aching joints, and oppressive sensations in the chest— are characteristically heavy and sluggish in nature and tend to block the flow of energy throughout the body. "Inner-dampness" is caused by excess consumption of liquor, tea, cold melons, and sweet, greasy foods. These impede spleen functions and cause symptoms of abdominal swelling, vomiting, and diarrhoea.

DRYNESS: Dryness belongs to the element Metal and dominates in autumn. Two types are distinguished: "cold-dryness" and "hot-dryness," depending on other conditions. Dry-excess easily injures the lungs, causing symptoms of heavy coughing, blood in the sputum, dry nose and throat, and pains in the chest. Dry-excess is also harmful to the body's fluid balance. "Inner-dryness" is caused by excessive loss of fluids due to too much sweating, vomiting, bleeding, or diarrhoea. Use of herbal medicines which induce sweating, vomiting, or purging of the bowels can also induce inner-dryness. Characteristic symptoms are dry, wrinkled, or withered skin, dry hair and scalp, dry mouth and cracked lips, dry stomach, and hard, dry stools.

FIRE: When any of the five excesses as described above become too extreme, they often transform to fire-excess. The symptoms are usually more intense forms of those associated with the original excess, plus symptoms of extreme heat-excess. "Inner-fire" is caused by excess emotional activity or by over-indulgence in food, drink, and sex. Violent anger, for example, often causes a sensation of heat rising from the upper abdomen, where liver-fire is raging. Too much strong food and drink causes fire to collect in the stomach; deep grief or passion will often cause it to rise in the lungs.

The Six Excesses which occur during the four seasons do not affect every person in the same way. Indeed, exceptionally healthy persons are not adversely affected by any of them. An "evil-excess" will attack the body only when and where it is weak and only when the protecting-qi is deficient somewhere along the surface of the body. One of the purposes of preventive medicine is to keep the body strong and resistent to such outside attacks.

Disease of the Six Excesses are most likely to occur under abnormal weather conditions, when the body is prepared for the dominant seasonal excess and suddenly faces an opposite force. Sudden cold spells in mid-summer, for example, often cause epidemics of influenza. Similarly, people who travel or move from a cold, dry place to a warm, damp climate are more vulnerable to invasion by local meteorological excesses than natives of the region.

The Seven Emotions are the major internal causes of disease in Chinese medical theory. Emotional activity is seen as a normal, internal, physiological response to stimuli from the external environment. Within normal limits, emotions cause no disease or weakness in the body. However, when emotions become so powerful that they are uncontrollable and overwhelm or possess a person, then they can cause serious injury to the internal organs and open the door to disease. It is not the intensity as much as the prolonged duration of an extreme emotion which causes damage. Diseases of the Seven Emotions are essentially psychosomatic in nature. While Western physicians tend to stress the psychological aspects of psychosomatic ailments, the pathological damage these ailments cause to the internal organs is very real indeed and is of primary concern to the Chinese physician.

Excess emotional activity causes severe yin-yang energy imbalances, wild aberrations in the flow of blood and qi blockages in the meridians, and impairment of vital organ functions. Extreme emotions, when permitted to dominate a person for too long, result in damage to the organs, allowing disease to enter the body from the outside or to develop from some mild, inherent weakness inside. Once physical damage has begun, it is insufficient to eliminate the offending emotion to effect a cure; the prolonged emotional stress will require physical action as well.

The Seven Emotions are joy, anger, anxiety, concentration, grief, fear, and fright. In excess, each of these emotions has debilitating effects on specific organs. They are described briefly below.

"When one is excessively joyful, the spirit scatters and can no longer be stored," stated the Chinese texts. Since the heart houses the spirit, excessive and prolonged joy—such as fits of uncontrollable laughter—injures the heart. It has already been noted that people who laugh a lot (Fire sound) are often found to have over-active hearts (Fire organ).

"If blood has a surplus, then there is anger." Quality and quantity of available blood are controlled by the liver, and anger is the emotion associated with it. An excess of rich blood in the system makes one prone to anger. It is commonly observed that ruddy, "full-blooded" people with flushed faces (blood-excess) are more prone than others to sudden fits of rage at the slightest provocation. Rather than burn itself out, anger feeds itself. It weakens the blood and injures the liver. This causes liver-qi to flare up even more uncontrollably, which in turn rushes upward and feeds the anger even more. Uncontrolled fits of anger are extremely injurious to the liver.

"When one feels anxiety, the qi is blocked and does not move." Anxiety injures the lungs, which control qi through breathing. Common symptoms of extreme anxiety are retention of breath, shallow and irregular breathing, and breathing only with the upper chest. The shortage of breath experienced during periods of anxiety is common to everyone. Anxiety also injures the lungs' coupled organ, the large intestine. For example, over-anxious people are highly prone to ulcerative colitis.

Over-concentration is said to harm the spleen, which houses the mind. This emotion refers to the type of obsessive fixation with the sort of problem which occupies one's mind from dawn to dusk. Such excessive, prolonged brooding impedes spleen and stomach functions, impairing digestion and causing abdominal pains.

Grief is not associated exclusively with one organ. Depending on its origin, grief can come to rest in either

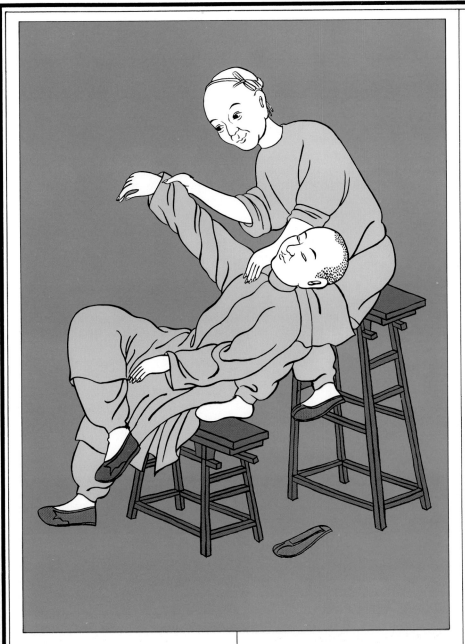

cited as the primary cause of dysentery. Stomach aches, vomiting, diarrhoea, and abdominal swelling are often attributed to too much "cold" or "cool" foods in the diet. Excessive indulgence in one of the five flavours associated with the Five Elements injures the associated organ. The various ailments caused by excess intake of alcohol are similar to those in the West.

Proper exercise is considered vital to maintaining health, and its absence is one of the miscellaneous causes of disease. Lack of physical exercise impairs health by making the flow of blood and energy sluggish. This accelerates the natural process of deterioration in the vital organs, muscles, and *qi*. On the other hand, excessive physical labour or fatigue will also promote weakness and disease in the body. "If there is exhaustion, the *qi* deteriorates."

Epidemics, serious wounds, insect and animal bites, worm infestation, penetrating poisons, and hereditary diseases are other factors which appear under "miscellaneous causes." Diseases which fall under this heading are the exception, not the rule.

In Chinese medical theory, all diseases have a definite cause, either internal or external in origin. Of the two, internal factors are more important because it is internal weakness which first permits invasion by external excess forces. A strong, healthy, well-balanced body and spirit will resist attack from even the most extreme environmental excesses. This again explains the important and repetitious stress in all Chinese medical texts on basic preventive care through diet, exercise, breathing, regulated sex, and preventive herbal prescriptions.

The relative balance among the body's vital energies and the environment's cosmic forces are the primary regulators of health and vitality. In the end, it boils down to a battle between "evil-*qi*" and "pure-*qi*." *The Internal Book of Huang Di* states, "where evil-*qi* gathers, it will cause weakness....When pure-*qi* is inside,

the heart, lungs, pericardium, or triple-warmer. It has a very debilitating effect on the body's store of *qi*.

"If the *qi* of the kidneys is weak, then one is prone to fear." The kidneys house the human attribute of will-power. When will-power is weak, one easily succumbs to fear. Excess fear injures the kidneys, and weak kidneys in turn arouse further feelings of fear. Again, the cycle of emotional excess and physical damage becomes a vicious circle. The phenomenon of involuntary urination during moments of intense fear has been observed often enough, demonstrating its association with the kidneys (and thus with its coupled organ, the bladder).

Fright is the other emotion not specifically related to only one organ. It is distinguished from fear by its sudden, unexpected nature. Fright primarily affects the heart, especially in its initial stages, but if it persists for some time, it becomes conscious fear and moves to the kidneys.

In addition to the meteorological and emotional causes of disease — which comprise the vast majority — the Chinese also acknowledge a variety of other causal factors for certain diseases. Excess food and drink or improper diet can cause a variety of ailments, with symptoms such as heartburn, constipation or irregularity, foul breath, and loss of appetite. Ingestion of rotten foods is

ABOVE Taking the pulse, *qie mai*, the initial diagnostic technique of both Chinese and Western medicine.

39

evil-*qi* cannot interfere with the body....When pure-*qi* prospers, evil-*qi* flees...When evil-*qi* is driven out, pure-*qi* grows." The beginning and end of Chinese medical theory is the concept of *qi* and its many manifestations, and it is *qi* that is manipulated in the practical applications of Chinese herbal medicine.

CHINESE DIAGNOSIS AND SYMPTOMOLOGY

Chinese diagnosis involves the reading of basic physical indicators of health and disease such as complexion, eyes, colour and texture of tongue and tongue fur, the patient's personal habits, pulse, and so forth. To this data, the physician applies the medical theories of disease to form a diagnosis and recommend a treatment. Neither the diagnosis nor the treatment remains static: the doctor must keep in close touch with the patient throughout the course of treatment and constantly review both diagnosis and treatment according to the derections taken by the disease. These directions are reflected in symptomatic changes. Herbal prescriptions are thus regularly revised according to the requirements indicated by the latest developments and symptoms.

Chinese physicians use four basic methods of diagnosis: interviewing, observing, listening, and feeling. Interviews take the form of comprehensive, and detailed dialogue between the doctor and patient. The interview must be well-organised and systematic, focusing on the major symptoms of the disease and background factors which may have contributed to its development. Above all, the interview must be objective and frank.

The order of business in such diagnostic interviews is first for the patient to describe the chief complaints and more obvious symptoms of his ailment. This is followed by an explanation of how, when, and where he first felt ill, followed by a description of the history of the illness from its onset right up to the day he visits the doctor, noting especially symptomatic changes, specific pains, and other manifestations unique to the ailment. Six indicators are emphasized during this part of the interview:

CHILLS AND FEVER: Intermittent fever and chills usually indicate an ailment which affects both the internal and external parts, or is moving from one to the other. Fever and thirst with no chills indicates an internal ailment, chills without fever reflects yang-deficiency, and fever without chills indicates an over-abundance of yang-energy. Other factors, such as what time of day chills and fever occur, further refine the reading of this indicator.

PERSPIRATION: The amount and viscosity of perspiration, when it occurs and on what parts of the body it appears, are the main questions regarding this sign.

STOOL AND URINE: Constipation accompanied by hard stools is a sign of "hot" and "solid" disease. Loose stools containing partially digested food indicates a "cold" and "empty" ailment. The presence of blood or mucus in the stool must also be reported. Scanty, dark urine reflects "heat-excess," while profuse, clear urine is a sign of "cold" and "empty" disease. Cloudy urine indicates "moist-heat excess."

FOOD, DRINK, AND TASTE: An inclination for hot drinks reflects a "cold" disease, while a preference for cold drinks and food indicates a "hot"-type disease. A revulsion towards drinking water is a sign of "moist" disease. The presence of a flat, bitter, sweet, or other dominant taste in the mouth must be reported. A strong desire for spicy, deep-fried foods or strange materials (such as dirt, candle-wax, coffee-grounds etc.) usually indicates the presence of parasites in the system.

SLEEP: Excessive sleep indicates yang-deficiency, while insomnia is a sign of poor circulation, excessive worry, or spleen-deficiency. Fitful sleep indicates emotional disturbance or over-indulgence in food and drink. Unusually early rising often indicates an over-active heart.

SEX, MENSTRUATION, AND PREGNANCY: For men, the vital questions in this area involve sexual vitality, impotence, incontinence, nocturnal emissions and spermatorrhoea, and frequency of coitus. For women, frequency of menstruation, its colour and texture, other vaginal discharges such as leukorrhoea, past pregnancies and/or abortions, childbirths, and frequency of coition are vital indicators of the nature of disease in the body.

In addition to the history of the specific disease based on the above indicators, a comprehensive past history of the patient himself is also taken. Besides stressing past illnesses, living habits, enviromental surrounding, allergies, and so forth, the general health history of the patient's family is also covered. In cases involving infants, the deaf and dumb, and others who are unable to conduct the interview for themselves, the relevant information is provided by the patient's spouse, parent, close family member, or friend.

Methodical visual observation of the patient is the second diagnostic technique used by traditional Chinese doctors. Changes in the body's skin colouring and form, tongue colour and tongue fur, eyes, secretions and excretions, all reflect the state of disease inside. First, the doctor notes the patient's mood and movements. If he is spirited and alert, with regular breathing and normal colouring, the illness is not yet serious and can be easily treated. If he is depressed and moody, with irregular breathing, wan complexion, and listless eyes, the disease has reached a serious stage and the treatment will be more complex. The colour and flesh-tone of a patient's facial complexion are direct indicators of pathological changes in the vital organs. The physician observes the patient's general physical condition by noting the way he walks, talks, sits down, lies, breathes, and moves his limbs.

One of the most important methods of observation-diagnosis is visual examination of the tongue. Such factors as muscular form and colour of the tongue and the colour and texture of the tongue fur reveal the empty-full nature of disease as well as its severity. Normal tongues are soft and moist, light-pink in colour and neither thick nor thin. If

Diagnosis Based On Examination Of The Tongue And Tongue Fur

Tongue colour and/of form	Tongue fur	Diagnosis
pale-white and weak	white, thin	qi and blood empty
pale-white; swollen and tender with teethmarks	white, thin	yang-empty
pale-white; swollen and tender	grey-black, slippery and moist	yang-weak; internal organs cold
pale-red; tender and jagged	no fur	qi-empty; yin-weak
pale-red	white, thin, slippery	external wind-cold
pale-red	white, thick, oily	indigestion; internal inflammation
pale-red moving	white with yellow traces	external evil-qi inward
pale-red already	yellow and thick centre; white, thin and slippery at edges	external evil-qi inside; stomach and intestines hot
bright-red	white, very thin	yin-empty; heat-excess
red, deep and jagged wrinkles	no fur	yin-weak; fluid-deficient
red	yellow, thin	heat-excess rising
red	yellow, oily	moist-heat excess
red	yellow, thick and dry	heat-excess deep inside
red	black, dry	heat-excess has injured yin
crimson	dark-yellow	heat-excess penetrated to nourishing-qi
dark-purple	dark-yellow, thin, dry	heat-excess penetrated to blood
light-purple and blood	white, slippery	internal cold; qi blocked

the tongue appears tight and shrivelled, the disease is of the "full" type; if it appears thick, porous, and tender, the ailment is of the "empty" type. A fat and swollen tongue indicates "moist-heat" excess inside the body. A light, pallid colour instead of the normal soft-pink indicates "blood-empty" and "qi-empty" disease, while a bright-red colour reflects "hot" and "full" disease. Normal tongues have a thin, white, clear fur coating that is neither too moist nor too dry. Disease in the body usually thickens this fur coating. A raw, white fur results from "cold" and "moist" disease, while a yellow fur indicates "hot" and "full" disease. In observing tongue-fur, care must be taken not to confuse symptomatic colour changes with residual colouring from food and drink. The accompanying chart gives a detailed account of the diagnostic indications of tongue structure, colour, and fur.

The listening technique includes examination by ear and stethoscope as well as by smell (one Chinese character for "hear" also means "smell"). The physician listens to the patient's speech, breathing, coughing, and to the sounds emanating from the visceral organs. He uses his nose to check the smell of the patient's body excretions, which helps to determine the nature and location of disease. "Empty" ailments are indicated by low, weak speech, shallow, weak-sounding respiration, and a weak, low-pitched cough. "Full" ailments are reflected in restless, confused speech, rapid and noisy breathing, and a heavy, loud cough. Examination of the internal organs by stethoscope is performed over the heart, lungs, and abdomen. The various sounds or murmurs made by the heart during various stages of heart beat, and the sounds produced by the lungs during inhalation and exhalation are all important diagnostic indicators of energy imbalances and dysfunction in those organs.

Tactile examination includes traditional Chinese pulse diagnosis and other manual methods such as massage and acupressure. In pulse diagnosis, the physician places his first three fingers along the radial artery of the patient's wrist, feeling for three special points. Light pressure on these points reveals three separate pulses, while heavy pressure reveals yet three different ones, a total of six pulses on each wrist. Each of the twelve pulses reflects the condition of one of the twelve vital organs. With skilled, sensitive fingers, the Chinese doctor can detect over thirty different pulse qualities on each of the twelve pulses. The pulse qualities—such as "floating," and "sunken," "weak," "bounding,"—indicate the condition of the related organ. Past, as well as current diseases sustained by the organ are revealed by this method. It may also indicate inherent weakness which may lead to disease in the future. Chinese pulse diagnosis is a delicate art, difficult to master and requiring many years of practice. Its proven ability to trace the sources and courses of disease in the vital organs—past, present and future—seems almost miraculous to those unfamiliar with the technique.

Other tactile techniques include light massage examination and palpitation of the internal organs. Massage reveals the temperature of the skin, flesh, and extremities, "full" and "hot" or "empty" and "cold" disease. Massaging the spinal column often indicates where a disease is located because the spinal nerves associated with the diseased organ will be knotted and tight to the touch. Certain vital points along the meridians, called "alarm points," will be tender and painful under acupressure when the related organ is diseased or weak. Palpitation involves applying finger and palm pressure to the body's surface directly over vital organs to check their consistency and tone. Similar to this method is percussion: the physician uses the middle finger of one hand to hit the mid-joint of the middle finger of the other hand, which is placed palm down over the organ. The resonance of this percussion indicates the condition of the organ below.

Determining the nature and location of disease is only the beginning of Chinese diagnosis. To treat patients effectively with herbal medicines, the physician must next make a "differential diagnosis" based on symptomology. Differential diagnosis determines in which direction the disease is moving and the nature of its symptoms. Symptoms sometimes seem to disappear during treatment. In actual fact, they have usually transformed and moved elsewhere, following, for better or worse, the course of the disease. Halting treatment at this juncture, when the disease is still inside, may permit the disease to recur at some time in the future. Continuing the same herbal treatment, when the symptoms and disease have already changed form, is not effective in the long run. Herbal prescriptions must be regularly adjusted to meet the ever-changing symptomatic situation. Since no two patients are exactly alike in their reactions to disease and to medications, differential diagnosis is vital to the successful application of Chinese herbal medicine in individual patients.

There are eight categories of *ba gang*, differential diagnosis: yin/yang, internal/external, cold/hot, and empty/full. These categories ultimately overlap, and all disease falls into one of the two great categories of yin and yang, according to the clinical manifestations of all the eight indicators. The principles of differential diagnosis are indispensable guides for prescribing herbal treatments which match the requirements of the disease and its symptoms.

Yin-yang designates whether the disease is primarily injuring the patient's yin- or yang-energy and whether to treat with yin or yang herbs. Based on the four diagnostic techniques, the general symptoms indicate yin or yang disease, as outlined below:

Internal-external indicators differentiate the site, extent, and seriousness of the disease, revealing in which direction it is moving. As diseases get worse, they tend to move inward toward the bones and vital organs. Movement towards the exterior usually indicates that the cure is working. Cold-hot manifestations

YIN-YANG DIAGNOSIS BASED ON THE FOUR DIAGNOSTIC METHODS

Diagnostic technique	Yang diagnosis	Yin diagnosis
interview	excess body heat and desire for coolness; great thirst and desire for fluids; constipation and hard stools; scanty, hot, dark urine	cold feeling and desire for warmth; lack of thirst and preference for hot drinks; loose stools; profuse, clear urine; flat taste in mouth; poor appetite
observation	flushed red face; bright eyes; nervousness; dry, cracked lips; bright-red tongue; thick, yellow tongue fur	pale, light complexion; drowsy eyes; fatigue; pale lips; pale, tender, swollen tongue; tongue fur white and slippery
listening and smelling	talkative and loud-mouthed; rapid, coarse breathing; heavy, foul-smelling excretia	soft, low voice; few words; shortness of breath; shallow breathing; light, raw-smelling excretia
feeling	fast, floating, heavy, slippery pulse; warm hands and feet; abdominal pain with aversion to applied pressure	slow, sunken, weak pulse; cold hands and feet; abdominal pain with desire for applied pressure to relieve cramps
NOTE	all symptomatic changes which stimulate vital organ functions belong to yang	all symptomatic changes which suppress vital organ functions belong to yin

are used to differentiate the nature of the disease itself, while empty-solid indicators reflect the nature and extent of the illness, as well as the body's resistence to the specific disease.

The following chart lists the broad indications drawn from the eight principles of differential diagnosis.

There are, of course, many different combinations of the above factors, and their manifestations are different for every patient and disease. The important point is to match the medications directly to the actual symptoms at hand, regardless of the original diagnosis. Some of the more common combinations of the eight principles are charted below.

Chinese diagnosis involves a three-step process: The four diagnostic techniques, (*si zhen*), are first employed to determine the general type, location, and cause of the disease. Next, differential diagnosis based on the eight principles, (*ba gang*), is applied to reveal to what

extent the disease has developed; in which direction it is moving and exactly how the symptoms are affecting the individual patient. Finally, based on the latest differential diagnosis, an herbal prescription is prepared which takes the body in the opposite symptomatic direction of the disease and redresses the energy imbalances caused by it. Regular re-evaluation of the data and diagnosis, followed by re-adjustment of the herbal formulas prescribed, continues until a complete cure is effected.

Having briefly covered the essential principles upon which traditional Chinese medicine is founded, we now return to the *ben cao* itself to see how this vast treasure-house of Chinese herbal knowledge is actually used in the practical application of Chinese herbal medicine.

The Eight Principles Of Differential Diagnosis

Principle	Major symptoms	Tongue and fur	Pulse	Treatment
yin	pale complexion; fatigue; shortness of breath; weak voice; loose stools profuse, clear urine	pale, tender; white, slippery fur	sunken; weak; slow	warming; tonifying
yang	flushed, red complexion; restlessness; loud voice; rapid, hard breathing; scant, dark urine; constipation and hard stools	bright-red; thick, yellow fur	floating; heavy; fast	cooling; sedative
internal	no independent symptoms; depends on hot/cold and full/empty indicators	changing	sunken	depends on hot/cold and full/empty indicators
external	fever and/or chills; aversion to wind and cold	normal colour; white, thin fur	floating	expel; induce perspiration
cold	aversion to cold; cold hands and feet; pale, white complexion; no thirst and preference for hot drinks; profuse, clear urine; loose stools	pale; white, slippery fur	slow	warming dispel cold
hot	aversion to heat; hot hands and feet; great thirst with preference for cold drinks; nervousness; scant, dark urine; hard stools	red; dry, yellow fur	rapid; bounding	cooling; edative
empty	weakness and fatigue; shortness of breath; low resistance; poor appetite; weight loss	thick, tender; little or no fur	weak; slow	tonifying
full	over-active body functions; restlessness; loud voice; coarse breathing; abdominal distention; scanty, dark urine; constipation	hard; thick fur	bounding	scatter and expel; purge

Common Combinations Of The First Principles Of Different Diagnosis

Combination	Major symptoms	Tongue and fur	Pulse
external-cold	fever and chill; no perspiration; head-and body-aches	normal colour; white, thin fur	floating; tight
external-hot	fever; head-ache; aversion to wind; intermittent perspiration	red; white or slightly yellow fur	floating; rapid
external-empty	aversion to wind; perspiration	pale	floating; slow
external-full	head-and body-aches; no perspiration	normal colour; white fur	floating; bounding
internal-cold	aversion to cold; no thirst; cold hands and feet; loose stools	white, slippery fur	sunken; slow
internal-hot	aversion to heat; great thirst; bloodshot eyes; fever; nervousness	red; yellow fur	rapid
internal-empty	weakness and fatigue; shortness of breath; aversion to talk; listless spirit; diarrhoea	pale-red; pale pale, thin fur	weak
internal-full	coarse breathing; perspiration on hands and feet; full feeling in abdomen; nervousness	hard; thick, yellow, dry fur	forceful; sliding

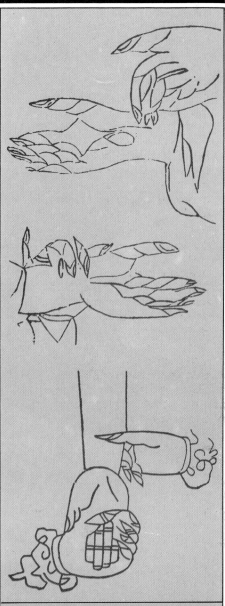

Pulsation and palpation techniques, TOP a doctor compares his pulse with that of his patient, and ABOVE for the right wrist of a female patient and BELOW the left wrist of a man. (below).

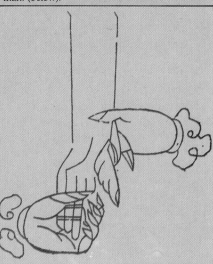

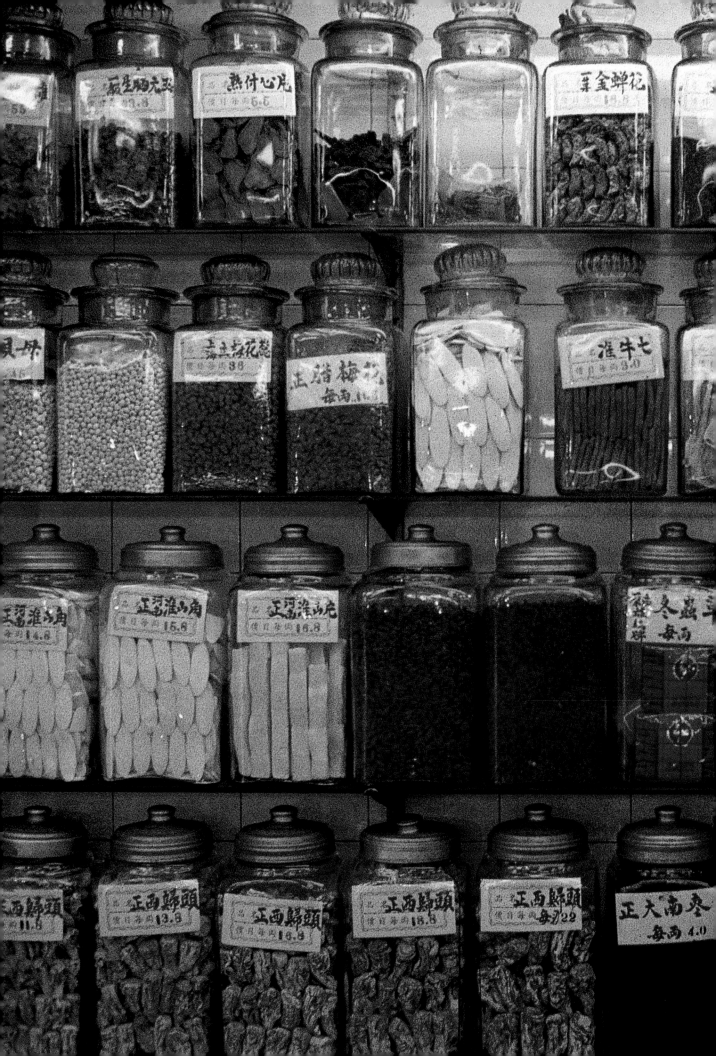

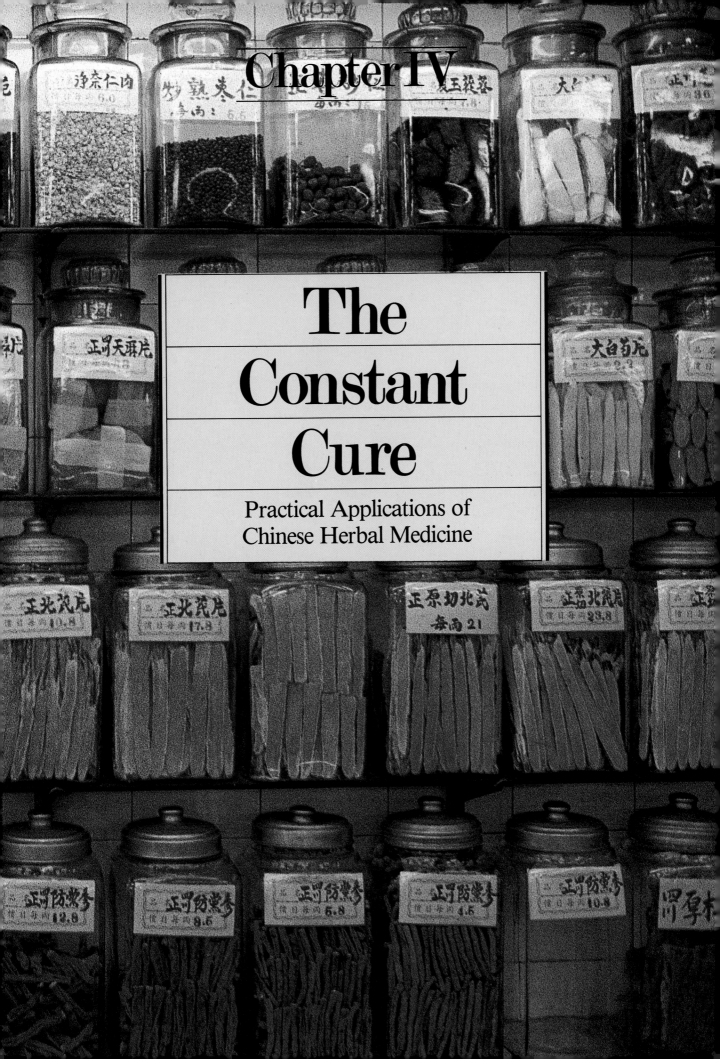

Chapter IV

The
Constant
Cure

Practical Applications of
Chinese Herbal Medicine

The theories of yin and yang and the Five Elements underpin the practical application as well as the principles and premises of Chinese herbal medicine. Just as causes, disease, and symptoms are all classified by their cosmological natures, so are herbal medicines classified. Items for herbal prescriptions are selected from the various categories to counteract the causes and to relieve the symptoms of disease.

GETTING THE RIGHT TOOL FOR THE JOB

The pathology of a disease and the pharmacology of the herbs used to cure it must match like lock and key throughout the entire course of treatment. The universal principles of yin-yang and the Five Elements are especially useful here because the same principles apply equally in plants and man, thereby providing a common theoretical framework for both human pathology and herbal pharmacology.

Differential diagnosis classifies all diseases by their symptoms into the broad categories of yin or yang. Chinese herbology similarly divides all herbal medicines into yin and yang categories. Employing the principles of opposites and relative balance, yin drugs are used for yang illnesses, and yang drugs are used to treat yin illnesses. The connections between symptoms and diseases, medications and effects, are outlined in a simple chart:

Symptoms	Disease	Medication	Desired effects
hot	yang	yin	cooling
cold	yin	yang	warming
full	yang	yin	sedate
empty	yin	yang	tonify
external	yang	yin	suppress
internal	yin	yang	elevate

Medicinal plants are first categorised by their Four Energies, *si qi*, and Five Flavours, *wu wei*. The Four Energies are hot, warm, cold, and cool, and they indicate the basic effect of the herb on the body. Hot and warm medications belong to yang, while cold and cool medications fall under the yin heading. In other words, those medications which have been proven over time to relieve the symptoms and cure the causes of hot/full/yang diseases are classified as cold or cool yin drugs. Those which relieve and cure cold/empty/yin illnesses are classified as hot or warm yang herbs. The distinction between hot and warm, cold and cool, is simply one of degree. Strong, robust patients can tolerate the more potent, faster-acting hot and cold medications. Weak and elderly patients are generally treated with the milder, slower-acting warm and cool drugs.

The principle of opposites applies in selecting medications according to the Four Energies. *The Internal Book of Huang Di* states, "If the disease is cold, heat it; if the disease is hot, cool it." And the *Pharmacopoeia of Shen Nong* agrees: "Cure cold diseases with warming medications; cure hot diseases with cooling medications." It is vital to properly match symptoms and treatments. If a patient displaying the symptoms of yang-excess (body heat, nervousness, thirst, flushed face, etc.) is treated with yang herbs, these symptoms would be quickly compounded and intensified until the yin-yang balance in his body is so upset that, in extreme cases, death might occur.

The Five Flavours of herbal drugs tie them to the theory of the Five Elements. The Five Flavours are hot, sour, bitter, sweet, and salty. The empirical evidence of the ages has shown that each of these five basic flavours indicates a specific pharmacological trait and specific pathological effect of the drug. The Five Flavours and their associations are described like this:
In addition, Chinese herbalists also distinguish a "plain" or "flat" flavour, i.e., no particular flavour, which acts similarly to hot and sweet herbs. In terms of the yin-yang balance, the hot, sweet, and plain flavoured herbs belong to yang, and the sour, bitter, and salty herbs belong to yin.

The Five Flavours are as important as the Four Energies in determining which medications suit the patient's condition. For example, patients who generally have insufficient fluid in the body should avoid using bitter herbs because they have a drying effect and would only aggravate the patient's fluid-deficiency. Similarly, people with energy-deficiency must avoid hot-flavoured medications because this category of herbs tends to scatter energy. The Five Flavours and Four Energies are thus considered together in selecting appropriate items for an herbal prescription.

Some herbs have the same energy classification but different flavours. Others may belong to the same flavour-group but have different energies. Examples of same energy, different flavour are fresh ginger (warm and hot), magnolia (warm and sour), and *Astragalus membranaceus* (warm and sweet). Examples of same flavour, different energy are mint (hot and cool), *Pinellia ternata* (hot and warm), and aconite (hot and hot). There are also herbs which possess several flavours and thus have several effects in the body: cinnamon is both hot and sweet in flavour, and *Rehmannia glutinosa* is both bitter and sweet. These distinctions are vital in the practical applications of Chinese herbal medicine and can become very complex. Many herbs are added to prescriptions solely to offset unwanted side-effects of other, more vital ingredients. Extensive clinical experience with a broad range of cases is required to learn the

Flavour*	Element	Related organ	Effects	Example
hot	metal	lungs; large intestine	induce sweat; balance *qi*; scatter blockage	fresh ginger
sweet	earth	stomach; spleen	digestive tonic; distribute nutrition	Chinese licorice
sour	wood	liver; gall bladder	binding; astringent; anti-pyretic	unripened plums
bitter	fire	heart; small intestine	drying; antidysenteric	bark of amur cork tree
salty	water	kidneys; bladder	softening; laxative; diuretic	algae and sea weed

*hot like ginger; sweet like sugar; sour like vinegar; bitter like lime; salty like salt

subtleties of selecting the right herbal tools for the job of curing a particular disease in a particular patient.

Two other important functional distinctions among herbal potions are those of ascending-descending and elevating-suppressing. Medications which cause energy to rise in the body are used against symptoms of descending energy. Medications which cause energy to descend are used in cases of uncontrolled ascending energy; this is also known as "quelling rebellious-*qi*". Elevating herbs tend to move upwards and scatter energy, while suppressing herbs move downward to gather and concentrate energy. Combining these functions, it is said that herbal potions which ascend and elevate in the system tend to move vital-energy up and out—for example, those which induce sweating or vomiting. They belong to yang. Herbs which descend and suppress tend to move vital-energy down and in—such as those which stop sweating or vomiting, purge the bowels, or suppress rebellious-*qi*. They belong to yin.

While each individual ingredient in an herbal prescription has a natural tendency to ascend and elevate or desend and suppress, it is the dominant net tendency of the entire prescription which determines how the entire mixture behaves in the body. For example, if items with a strong tendency to ascend and elevate are mixed with an equal quantity of items with a weak tendency to descend and suppress, the entire herbal mixture will tend to ascend and elevate energy. Both the doctor and the herbalist must be thoroughly familiar with the basic nature, dominant tendency, natural affinity, and general effects of every item in the *ben cao* in order to prepare effective herbal prescriptions. The correlations among the essential energies, flavours, directions and effects of herbal drugs are summarised in the chart below:

The broad division of herbal medicines according to their Four Energies, Five Flavours, and general directions is only the first step in tailoring herbal prescriptions to the

Yang		Yin	
ESSENTIAL ENERGY			
tonify yang	hot	cold	tonify yin
purge cold	warm	cool	purge cold
ESSENTIAL FLAVOUR			
scatter balance *qi* binding	hot	sour	astringent;
digestive tonic; distribution	sweet	bitter	drying; concentrating
move fluid; diuretic	plain	salty	soften; laxative
ESSENTIAL DIRECTION			
upward-moving *qi*-nurturing *qi*-suppressing	ascend	descend	downward-moving;
outward-moving; scattering	elevate	suppress	inward-moving; concentrating

precise requirements of the disease and patient. Medicinal plants with the same essential energy, flavour, and direction often have widely different uses in application. This depends upon their natural affinities (*gui jing*) for various parts of the body. Once the correct categories of herbal medication have been determined, the doctor must select items from among those categories which have natural affinities for the parts of the body he wants to treat. For example, excess heat in the lungs and excess heat in the liver are both treated with yin herbs which cool, descend, and suppress and fall into the sour, bitter, or salty flavour categories. However, the specific items chosen for the lung prescription are not the same as those chosen for the liver prescription, because their organ affinities are different. Furthermore, during the course of disease, "evil-*qi*" may move from the originally infected organ to another one, in which case the herbal prescription must be adjusted to include herbs with affinities for the newly infected organ. Like everything in Chinese herbal medicine, the natural affinities of the myriad herbs in the *ben cao* have been gradually established

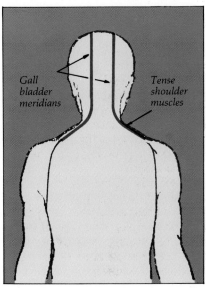

Gall bladder meridians

Tense shoulder muscles

through centuries of trial-and-error experimentation and inductive reasoning.

The natural affinities of herbs may also be determined by using the Five Elements system. Colour, aroma, and flavour of the herbal items are used as guides in this system of identification:

An herbal medication with a natural affinity for an organ not only affects that organ directly, but also affects the entire meridian connected to the organ. A drug's organ affinity

RIGHT Diagram shows the gall bladder meridians and their relationship to the shoulder muscles — hence the treatment of the gall bladder or liver to relieve tension.

Herbal drug			Five elements identity	Organ	affinity
Colour	Flavour	Aroma	Element	Yin	Yang
blue/green	sour	pungent	Wood	liver	gall bladder
red	bitter	scorched	Fire	heart	small intestine
yellow	sweet	fragrant	Earth	spleen	stomach
white	hot	rank/raw	Metal	lungs	large intestine
black	salty	rotten/putrid	Water	kidneys	bladder

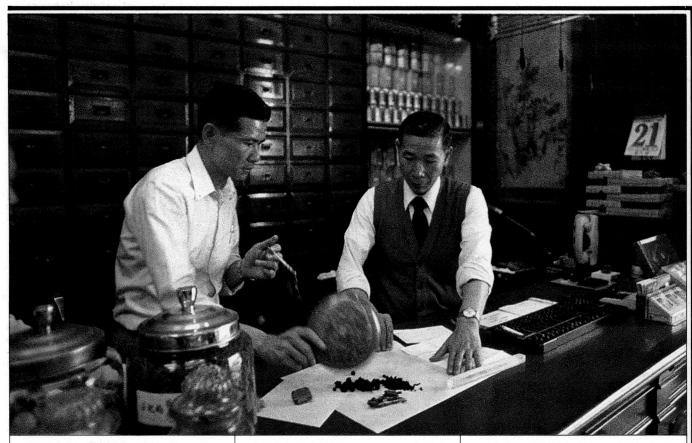

therefore indicates not only which organ it goes to, but also which other parts of the body are affected by it. For example, there are no vital organs located in the head, yet herbal prescriptions are very effective in curing headaches of all types. How? If it is a frontal headache, herbs with affinity for the stomach are used. The stomach meridian passes up through the face and forehead, which therefore benefit from the vital-energy flowing along the stomach meridian. If the headache is in the back of the head, it can be relieved by treating the gall bladder because the gall bladder meridian runs up the back of the neck and head. A simple glance at a meridian chart indicates which organs must be treated to effect relief of pain on any part of the body.

There are two other functional distinctions among herbal medications which must be considered: tonify-sedate and moisten-dry. These distinctions relate to the full/empty symptomology of disease. *The Internal Book of Huang Di* states, "If there is fullness, sedate it; if there is emptiness, tonify it." Tonic herbs are those which tonify the vital primordial energies, *bu yuan qi*, improve

the tone of bodily tissues, and eliminate symptoms of weakness and fatigue. Sedative herbs are those which have a calming, soothing effect and suppress excess evil-*qi*. "Full" symptoms—energy-excess, over-activity —are thus treated with sedative, calming, medications, and "empty" symptoms—energy-deficiency, under-activity—are treated with tonic, stimulating, medication. Again, these distinctions indicate the general type and general effects of herbal drugs. For specific application to specific organs, natural affinities must be considered in selecting the right herbal tools.

In curing full/empty disease, not only does the diseased organ itself

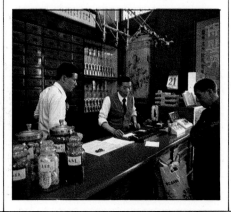

have to be treated, but also the main organ affecting, or being affected by, the diseased organ. The mother-son relationship applies, and the rule is: If the organ is "empty," tonify its mother; if the organ is "full," sedate its son. For example, if the heart, Fire, is empty, then the liver, Wood, must be tonified as well as the heart because Wood is mother to son Fire, and a tonified mother generates a more tonified son. On the other hand, if the heart is full, then the stomach as well as the heart should be sedated because Earth is son to mother Fire, and sedation relieves the stomach, Earth, of excess generation by the full heart, Fire.

Herbs have an essentially drying or moistening nature as well. Those herbs high in oil and water content are considered moisturising and are used against disease of dry-excess and fluid deficiency. Drying herbs are usually devoid of oil and moisture and are used to absorb damp-excess in the body.

Based on these details, we can delineate eight basic approaches to the treatment of disease using Chinese herbs:

PERSPIRATION METHOD: The Chinese

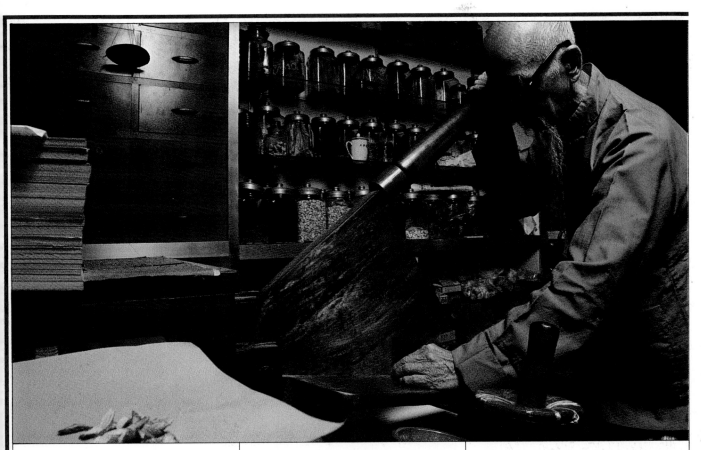

term literally means "to release externally." It is used against ailments of external exposure. Herbs which induce perspiration are divided into warm and cool types: the warm inducers are used in wind-cold ailments; the cool inducers are applied to wind-heat ailments.

EMETIC METHOD: Emetic herbs induce vomiting and are used for "full" and/or acute ailments of the upper parts of the body. All drugs which induce vomiting fall into this category. They remove pathogenic matter from the stomach and small intestine.

PURGATIVE METHOD: This method lubricates the large intestine to induce loose, "hot" stools, which bring out the "full-heat" accumulated inside. There are two types: purgatives and laxatives. Purgatives exert a strong action and are appropriate for acute illnesses in patients who are still strong and otherwise healthy. Laxatives have a milder, slower lubricating action and are best suited for chronic ailments and weak, elderly patients.

NEUTRALISER METHOD: This method utilises the neutralising, balancing effects of herbal drugs. It is often employed when a disease is on the move between internal and external locations. It is particularly effective against liver diseases which have a disruptive effect on other organs.

STIMULATION METHOD: This method is also called "warming." These drugs warm the interior to dispel cold, tonify yang-energy, and stimulate circulation of energy and blood. The yang herbs used in this method generally stimulate organ functions and eliminate cold-qi. They are also well suited for any type of qi-deficient ailment.

HEAT-CLEARING METHOD: The

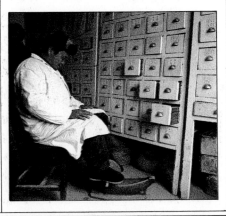

cooling yin medications used in this method clear up fever, reduce body temperature, stimulate salivary glands, and detoxify the system. There are a wide variety of heat-clearing herbs, and they are used against a broad spectrum of ailments. They all have the general effect of cooling the body's heat-excess and eliminating toxins.

DEFLECTION METHOD: This group of drugs is used in cases of stagnation, accumulation, congestion, etc. They tend to dispel, re-channel, and correct energy imbalances, and to loosen accumulated moisture such as sputum. They are divided into five types: energy-correcting; blood-correcting; digestion-promoting; sputum-liquefying; and moisture-converting.

TONIC METHOD: Tonics are used to treat cases classified as "empty", indicating a deficiency, and to supplement imbalances between yin and

OPPOSITE: A typical herbal medicine store where remedies are often sold by weight (top) and ingredients are sliced (above) or ground (left) into powder.

yang in blood and *qi*. There are four types: yang-nurturing; yin-nurturing; energy-nurturing; and blood-nurturing. Yang-nurturing tonics are used against yang-energy deterioration and "cold-empty" ailments. Yin-nurturers are prescribed for yin-energy deficiency and damage to yin-energy caused by fever, heat, dryness and other yang excesses. Energy-nurturing herbs are suitable for general convalescence, fatigue, and weakness. Blood-nurturing tonics supplement and nourish the blood and are used in all cases of blood-deficiency, such as anemia, post-natal blood loss, malnutrition, etc.

The classification of all herbal ingredients according to their essential natures and primary effects is the starting point for mixing effective herbal prescriptions. The herbal distinctions of Four Energies and Five Flavours, ascend-descend, elevate-suppress, tonify-sedate, and moisten-dry all correspond to equivalent distinctions in diagnosis and symptomology. Applying the universal principles of yin-yang and the Five Elements as well as the specific natural affinities of each herb, Chinese physicians use the basic herbal classifications to select the right tools for the job of curing disease by matching herbal pharmacology to disease pathology.

HOW THE HERBS ARE MIXED FOR THE PATIENT

Even today, the typical Chinese herbal medicine shop conveys a feeling that little has changed for thousands of years. Rows and rows of worn wooden drawers, a simple teak counter, crude balance scales, the everpresent abacus, choppers and grinders identical to those depicted in the ancient scrolls, and, of course, the age-old varieties of herbs themselves. Why, Western physicians may wonder, don't they modernise the ancient art of herbal healing? Why don't they refine and purify the crude herbs, extract and concentrate their active ingredients, and produce modern medications in capsules and ampules? The answer is that the modern Western way is not necessarily nature's way, and nature's way, which never changes, is the way the

Chinese have been following since the early beginning of herbal medicine. It is also the way that herbal medicine works most effectively.

Take, for example, the Chinese herb *ma huang*, (*Ephedra sinica*). The roots and stems contain up to one percent of the alkaloid, ephedrine, which is the world's most effective preventive for bronchial asthma. This herb has now become scarce and quite expensive in Asia because the Western pharmaceutical industry buys up most of the available supply to refine the "modern" drug ephedrine from it. Refined, concentrated ephedrine brings immedi-

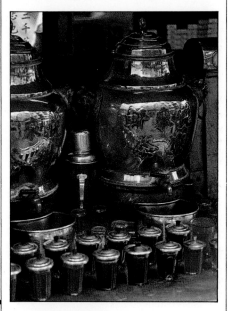

ate relief to those who suffer from bronchial asthma, but not only is the cost of the drug high, but so is the cost to the body: in its refined, Western form, ephedrine over-stimulates the heart muscle, causing palpitations and hypertension; it raises the blood-pressure considerably; and it induces a general state of nervous sensitivity. Obviously, such side-effects are exhausting in the long run and intolerable for patients with high blood-pressure or weak hearts.

The Chinese, however, use *ma huang* in its crude, natural form. While the effects are slower, there are no ill side-effects. The drug, in its natural state, is more suitable for gradual absorption into the metabolism of the body because the active ingredient, ephedrine, is accompanied by other natural ingredients in the plant. These act as metabolic buffers and prevent the shocks to the system caused by concentrated chemicals. Using crude herbs, the Chinese physician has the option to select not only the appropriate ingredients but also the appropriate method of preparing them for each individual patient. The traditional methods of mixing herbal prescriptions permit the herbalist to balance precisely and tune carefully the net effects of the prescription, according to the doctor's instructions. These methods of mixing and administering herbal medications are therefore every bit as important as the ingredients themselves.

To be sure, some progress has been made in recent years in China in producing refined, concentrated medications from crude herbs, mostly for relief of common ailments such as colds, fevers, indigestion, etc. Western medical technology is particularly helpful in this new aspect of herbal pharmaceutics, but on the whole this field of development is still in its infancy. The overwhelming majority of both practitioners and patients revere the traditional time-tested ways, and it seems likely that they will be supplanted very slowly by modern methods. That is why little has

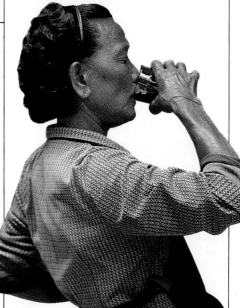

LEFT Herbal tea, one of the basic tonics of Chinese medicine. OPPOSITE: Roots, deer antlers, dried sea-horses and horns are among the more exotic tonics and aphrodesiacs.

changed in Chinese herbal shops for thousands of years.

Chinese herbal prescriptions are written up by the attending physician in the clinic, then taken by the patient to a Chinese herbalist, who expertly prepares the mixture. When the prescription takes the form of broth, tea, wine, or powder, the mixed ingredients are taken home and prepared for consumption by the patient. Pills, pastes, and other special forms must be prepared at the shop by the herbalist and usually require several days.

The actual form an herbal prescription takes depends upon the nature of the herbs used, the nature of the disease to be treated, and the patient's own physical constitution. Some herbs, for example, are only effective when ground to a talc-fine powder and mixed into pills, while others must be boiled or steamed to become medically active. On the other hand, some herbal ingredients can be used in many different forms, such as in pills for internal use as well as in pastes for external use. The various methods of preparing prescriptions differ in their concentrations of active ingredients and in their rates of absorption and distribution in the body. Weak or elderly patients are given gentler preparations which are absorbed slowly, while more robust patients can tolerate the stronger, faster-acting forms. Here is a brief description of the eight traditional methods of mixing herbal medications.

BROTH: This is the oldest and most common method of mixing and ingesting herbal prescriptions. The main advantages of this method is that the ingredients are absorbed quickly after ingestion and take effect immediately. The herbs are placed in a clean, earthenware cooking vessels with 3-4 cups of water, covered

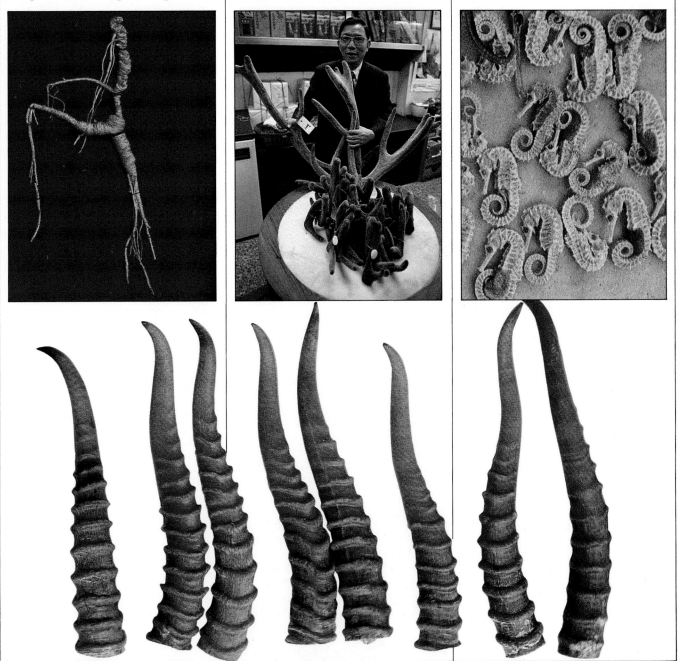

tighly, and boiled until nearly half of the liquid has evaporated. The amount of water, boiling time, and heat intensity all depend upon the type of herbs used. Fragrant, aromatic drugs such as mint, rose-buds, and cardamom are boiled for a short time over low heat. Mineral-derived ingredients, however, must be finely ground and first boiled alone over intense heat before the remaining herbs are added and the heat is turned down. Tonic prescriptions, which usually contain animal-derivatives, are boiled with much water over a low flame for a long time. Some ingredients must be wrapped in a cheese-cloth pouch to prevent irritating fibres from entering the broth.

After boiling, the broth is strained through cheese-cloth and divided into two or three portions, to be ingested between meals, when the stomach is empty and able to absorb quickly.

A related technique is to place the ingredients in a small covered clay or ceramic bowl with only a little water and steam the entire bowl in a steamer. This extracts a concentrated liquid known as "medicine dew." It is strong and fast-acting. Ginseng is often prepared this way by itself.

When fresh rather than dried herbs are available, "medicine-juice" can be extracted by mashing the herbs with a little water and squeezing out the juice. Fresh ingredients are stonger and more active than dried ones.

PILLS: Chinese herbal pills are made by grinding all the ingredients to a talc-fine powder, adding a binder such as honey, water, or beeswax, then rolling the mixture by hand into round pills. Size varies from that of buck-shot to large marbles, depending upon the strength required by the prescription. To ensure gradual, even absorption and the constant presence of the medication in the system, most pill prescriptions require the patient to take fifteen to twenty little pills three or four times a day. Herbal pills are slow-acting and gentle. They are used for treating long-standing, chronic ailments. This method is also preferred when the prescription includes strong, poisonous drugs, because absorption is

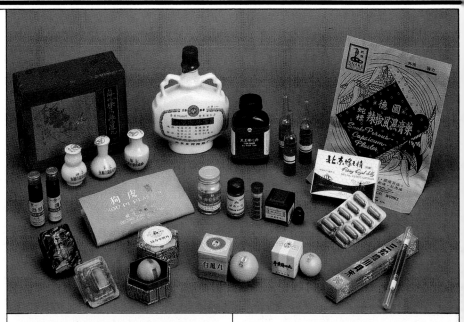

slow and gradual enough for the body to tolerate the toxins. Four varieties of pills are made from powdered herbs:

Honey pills: Honey-based pills are made by mixing all the powders with honey until smooth, rolling the dough-like mixture into long thin tubes, pinching off the amount required, and rolling it into pills between the thumb and fingers. The honey must first be boiled and skimmed to remove impurities so that the pills do not spoil in storage. Honey absorbs slowly in the stomach and small intestine and is itself a yin-tonic medication. Thus, honey pills are prescribed for long-term weaknesses and chronic ailments in which gradual but constant tonification is desirable.

Flour-paste pills: Rice or wheat flour is mixed with water to form a dry paste, to which the powdered herbs are added. The dough is formed into pills as above. These are used primarily in cases of stomach and intestinal ulcers, which cannot tolerate direct contact with potent herbal medications. The flour-paste acts as a digestive buffer while the medications are gradually dissolved and absorbed. The consistency and proportion of flour-paste is a vital factor in the efficacy of this type of pill.

Water pills: This method utilises the adhesive, sticky properties inherent to certain herbs in order to form pills. Since most of the water is removed in

the process and no other binder or buffer added, such pills absorb rapidly and act fast.

A large, round flat basket made of finely-woven bamboo is first sprinkled well with water. The powdered herbs are then sprinkled onto the inner surface, and the whole basket is rolled about in a circular motion. As the moisture activates the adhesive elements in the powders, small pills begin to form in the basket as it is rolled about. More water and powder are gradually sprinkled on until the correctly sized pills are formed.

Wax pills: Wax pills are made by using a binder of beeswax. They absorb very slowly, usually in the small intestine. Beeswax is used when highly toxic ingredients such as mercury or aconite appear in the prescription. This insures the slowest, most gradual rate of absorption possible.

After pills have been formed, they are sometimes coated with another single, pure ingredient. This is called "putting on the clothing." There are three purposes for this over-coat: sometimes a single ingredient from the prescription is set aside and put on last as an over-coat to insure that it dissolves and absorbs first; over-coats are sometimes added to prevent dampness and bugs from getting into the pills; and sometimes they are added to bitter prescriptions to make the flavour more palatable and the pills easier to eat.

PASTE: Pastes are prepared for both internal and external use. For internal use, the herbal ingredients are slowly boiled with water until a thick soup is formed. Water is continuously added and boiled off until a smooth, viscous texture is achieved. This is filtered to remove sediment and impurities, returned to the pot, and very slowly cooked until all water has evaporated, leaving a thick, smooth paste. To this paste honey or melted rock crystal sugar is added for flavour and to facilitate metabolism in the system. These concoctions may be stored in sealed jars in a cool, dry place. They are generally prescribed for chronic ailments and tonic use.

Pastes are most commonly used for external forms of herbal treatment and are of two types: "medicine-paste" and "paste-medicine." Medicine-paste is produced by mixing the powdered herbal ingredients in a base of animal fat, yellow vaseline, or vegetable oil to form an ointment. This is used as a balm for skin diseases, abscesses, etc. Paste-medicine is made by boiling the herbs until thick and sticky, skimming the oil from the surface and removing the sediment from the bottom, then adding lead or mercuric oxide and white vaseline until a sticky paste is formed. This paste is spread like butter onto a piece of cloth or wax-paper and taped tightly over the injured area for eight to twelve hours. These herbal poultices penetrate the skin to relieve ailments such as arthritis, rheumatism, twists and sprains, "wind-dampness" in joints and sinews, pain and numbness in muscle, and spinal ailments of all types. They are usually highly effective both in relieving symptomatic pain and effecting long-lasting cures for all such ailments. Patients with overly-sensitive skin must be careful using herbal poultices.

DAN MEDICATIONS: The Chinese character *dan* has been closely associated with Taoist alchemy and Chinese medicine for millennia. It literally means "the pill of immortality" or "elixir of life." These medications can resemble pills, powders, or chunks of metallic alloy, depending upon the ingredients. They generally contain very potent or toxic mineral derivatives, which originally were thought to contain the essential secret ingredients to immortality. Hence, the label *dan* is often attached to medications employing such ingredients. They are used for a wide variety of ailments and are highly potent.

MEDICINE-WINE: Medications steeped for a long time in strong liquor form "medicine-wine." It has the advantages of not spoiling in storage, easy ingestion, and fast action. However, since the liquor used must be quite strong, medicine-wine should not be used by patients who cannot tolerate alcohol or for ailments which preclude use of liquor. The most potent form of medicine-wine is called "Spring-Wine" because it contains ingredients which nurture sexual vitality.

The herbs are coarsely cut or left whole, put in large bottles or crocks, covered completely with a strong liquor, sealed, and stored for at least half a year. Today, brandy—especially fine French cognac—is highly favoured among Chinese connoisseurs for making Spring-Wine. When ready, the liquor is filtered and sweetened with rock crystal sugar for flavour and easier metabolism. One to two ounces should be drunk before retiring at night, more in cold weather and less in hot weather.

In ancient times, herbs were sometimes added directly to fermenting rice, so that they would ferment along with the rice to produce an herbal wine. This method is rarely used today because of difficulty in measuring dosages and controlling the fermenting process.

GUM: Gums are made from animal parts such as skin, bones, flesh, shells, and horns. They are mainly used in tonic preparations for patients suffering from weakness, fatigue, lassitude, and general lack of vitality. The dried hides of wild donkeys, tiger bones, tortoise shells, and stag-horns are common items for making gums. The ingredients are scraped clean of excess dried flesh and sinew, washed well, and placed in a pot with water. They are slowly simmered for a whole day and night, strained of sediment, simmered again with more water, strained, and simmered once more, until a thick, viscous liquid remains in the bottom of the pot. This is strained again and returned to the pot until all remaining water evaporates, leaving a gluey, translucent residue. When the residue cools, it achieves the texture of gum rubber and is cut into squares for use.

FERMENTATION: With this method, powdered herbs are mixed with flour and water and kneaded into dough. The dough is formed into balls and set aside to ferment. Such medications are used mostly for diseases of the stomach and spleen because fermentation with flour gives the entire prescription a natural affinity for those organs. Fermented prescriptions also promote digestion.

Such methods of preparing herbal prescriptions have stood the test of time. Ingredients are used in their natural forms, mixed with appropriate natural buffers, binders, and metabolic catalysts, and prepared in such a way that the body absorbs, distributes, and metabolises them at a rate suitable to the individual patient and his ailment, and appropriate dietary advice is always given

LEFT Medicinal or tonic wines, some of which are boosted with other remedial ingredients. OPPOSITE: A tiny selection of the vast modern-day pharmacopoeia of Chinese medicine.

53

along with the medications. Western medications, prepared and pre-packaged according to patent formulas, are not so readily tailored to the individual requirements of each patient. So common were personal herbal prescriptions by the time of the Ming dynasty, that in one novel of that era, the *Jin Ping Mei* ("Golden Lotus"), herbal prescriptions sometimes even appear in verse! This is one indication of how pervasive the use of herbal medicine has been in Chinese society.

PREVENTIVE AND CURATIVE MEDICINE

In ancient China, the primary purpose of herbal medicine was to prevent disease. Doctors were retained to ·keep families healthy and were held personally accountable whenever preventive efforts failed. A physician who had to wait for the onset of obvious signs and symptoms of disease before treating the problem was considered inferior. In the *Internal Book of Huang Di*, the Yellow Emperor's chief medical adviser states the point succinctly:

To administer medicines to diseases which have already developed and to suppress revolts which have already developed is comparable to the behaviour of those persons who begin to dig a well after they have become thirsty, and of those who begin to make their weapons after they have already engaged in battle. Would these actions not be too late?

Preventive medicine involves two basic approaches: the patient must cultivate proper personal habits of health and hygiene, and the physician must detect diseases to which the patient is prone and treat his vulnerable condition before disease strikes. The first approach includes such measures as proper diet, plenty of exercise, proper breathing, regulated sex life, and other daily preventive routines. Changes in season and weather must be met by appropriate adjustments in diet and other routines so that the optimum relative balance of energies within and without the body is maintained.

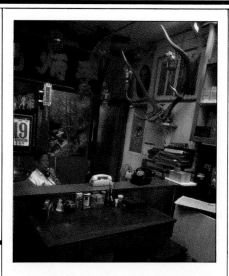

This personal, daily approach to preventive care is especially effective in preventing chronic and degenerative diseases from developing. It also raises one's general level of health, vitality, and resistance to infective diseases.

The latter preventive approach depends upon the physician's skill in reading the subtle signs of pre-clinical symptomology. Indicators such as a certain way of walking or talking, nervous habits, timbre of voice and breathing, emotional changes, dietary preferences, etc. often reflect a patient's vulnerability to certain forms of disease long before they strike. If the conditions which make the body vulnerable are corrected early enough, disease is prevented.

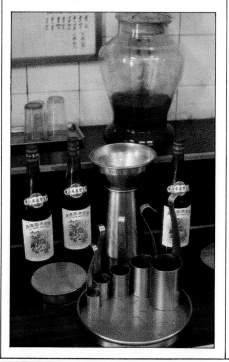

Pulse diagnosis generally reveals weaknesses in a patient's vital organs long before they become critical and permit disease to develop. Such weaknesses manifest themselves as abnormalities in the pulse of the affected organ. When discovered, they are immediately treated with appropriate herbal prescriptions and/or acupuncture. If the affected organs are too weak, or the detection of weakness comes too late, preventive treatment with herbs may need to continue for life in order to avoid serious disease. On the other hand, when the weak conditions are corrected and the pulse abnormalities and other pre-clinical symptoms disappear, the treatment may be discontinued.

The Chinese have always been concerned about their progeny, and one of the main purposes of preventive medicine is to strengthen the genetic plasma passed on to their offspring. Healthy, robust parents usually beget healthy, robust children. And children born healthy and robust go through life with less disease, greater vitality, and healthier minds. By keeping themselves in optimum health through preventive care, especially around the time of conception, the Chinese continually seek to improve their genetic stock. This no doubt contributes to the great tenacity and vitality the Chinese race has demonstrated throughout its long history.

Curative medicine is used when preventive medicine has failed or been ignored, thereby permitting disease to develop. It is also used in cases of virulent infectious disease, serious wounds, traumatic injuries, and other problems which defy preventive medicine. Curative herbal concoctions relieve the symptoms of disease by producing opposite symptomatic changes in the body. They cure the causes of disease by redressing the energy imbalances and tonifying the weak organs which permit disease to develop.

Chinese herbal cures may take a long time, but results often last a long time. If followed up with proper preventive care, the cures are usually permanent.

In applying curative herbal medication, it is vital not only to get the right tools for the job but also to be

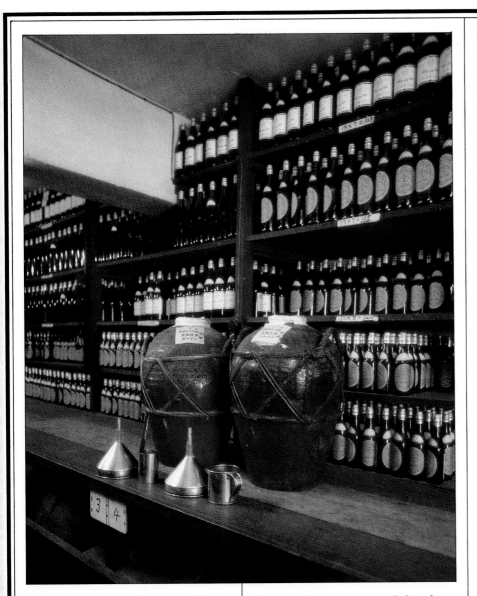

perhaps a bit envious of, their amorous behaviour, the goat-herd observed the horny animals carefully for a few weeks. He noted that whenever they ate from a certain patch of weeds, their promiscuous proclivities became pronounced for several hours thereafter. One thing led to another, and before long Chinese herbalists discovered *Epimedium sagittatum*, one of the strongest herbs for male potency in the entire *ben cao*. They called it *yin yang huo*—"horny goat weed".

This remarkable herb seemed custom-made by nature for the flagging male libido. Its strong, stimulating affinity for the supra renal glands—"kidney-glands" in Chinese—promote increased secretions of male hormones almost immediately. Recent research has shown that sperm count and semen density increase substantially during the first few hours after ingestion of this herb. In addition, it expands the minutest capillaries as well as the major vessels of the circulatory system, permitting hormone-enriched blood to penetrate the body's finest, most sensitive tissues. Improved circulation of fortified blood eliminates fatigue and multiplies available energy. Expansion of blood vessels induces a proportionate decrease in blood pressure, making the herb safe for those who need it most. And by flooding the brain with hormone-rich blood, sensitivity to tactile, visual, olfactory, and other forms of nervous stimulation is greatly amplified as well.

Tonics are the most interesting—and by far the most expensive—items in the Chinese pharmacopoeia. They are directly linked to longevity because of their proven power to promote vital-hormone production—the "vital-essence" of Chinese medical argot. The use of tonic herbs which increase sexual vitality combined with the practice of sexual techniques which preserve the vital-essence is an original and very old method of *yang sheng*, "nurturing-life". Only in recent decades has Western medical

OPPOSITE Deer antlers, used in powdered form as a tonic and aphrodesiac, adorn a druggists store, along with tonic wine measures (below) ABOVE Bottles and ceramic jugs of tonic wine.

effective at the right time. If the doctor misreads a symptom and prescribes the wrong medication, the condition is only compounded. Patients must consult the attending physician often enough for symptomatic changes to be analysed and herbal prescriptions adjusted accordingly. The doctor must follow the disease's development carefully and time his treatments so that they are always antagonistic to the major symptoms. Any side-effects or unexpected reactions must be promptly reported by the patient, and his diet and other daily routines adjusted and timed to the requirements of the cure. For example, when using mountain varnish (*Panax notoginseng*) internally, the patient must avoid beans, seafoods, and cold drinks of all kinds during the treatment because these items neutralise

the curative properties of this drug. Finally, the herbal treatment must be followed scrupulously according to the doctor's instructions from beginning to end. Some chronic ailments require months or even years of herbal treatment before they are thoroughly eliminated, and many patients sacrifice their chance for a permanent cure by becoming impatient and giving up the treatment too soon.

TONICS: THE LEGEND OF THE GOAT

Once there was a goat-herd in ancient China who noticed that several of his billy-goats were especially randy, often mounting their mates many times in a brief span of time. Curious about, and science discovered the fundamental connection between hormone production and the aging process.

The role of tonics in Chinese herbal medicine is best illustrated by the modern example of Yang Sen, the vigorous general from Sichuan who died in Taipei only a few years ago. He attained the ripe old age of 98, only three years short of the 101-year life-span of the great Sun Simiao, whose Taoist theories he practiced.

Yang Sen had always been interested in herbal medicines in his native Sichuan, where the best Chinese herbs grow. While still a young man, he began using tonics and other preventive herbs. He was known as a fierce fighter, an insatiable lover, and a man with a great zest for life. By the time he and his entourage arrived in Taiwan in 1949, he already had numerous wives and concubines and countless children to his name.

After retiring from military duty, Yang Sen became active in sports and physical education. He served as director of the Taiwan Sports Federation as well as the Taiwan Mountain Climbing Association. In the latter role, he led an annual climb to the 12,000-feet peak of Jade Mountain, the highest in Taiwan, and invariably left most of his much younger climbing companions panting and puzzled far down the trail. He continued this practice right to the year of his death. In fact, he had planned to celebrate his 100th birthday on the peak of Jade Mountain.

Why did Yang Sen possess more vigour than men half his age? He followed the Taoist "Way of Long-Life", including the sexual "Way of Yin and Yang". He used medicine-wine tonics to nurture his vital-energy and vital-essence and followed a strict regimen of physical exercise, always early to bed and early to rise. His foods were as carefully selected for potency and energy as were his herbs. And he cultivated the Way of Yin and Yang: he engaged in frequent and vigorous sexual intercourse with infrequent emission of semen, constantly building up and storing vital-essence. An extremely wealthy man, Yang Sen could well afford the expensive tonic herbs he favoured in and the young mistresses he kept. Every three to five years he sought

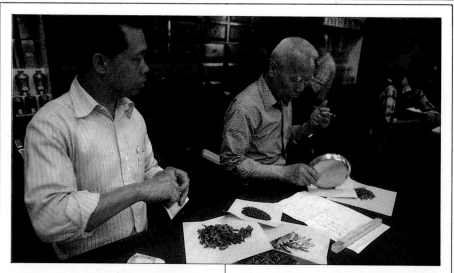

out a new partner, offering generous terms and stating only two requirements—that she be young and healthy and that she practise the Way of Yin and Yang with him for a few years. In this way he remained physically, mentally, and sexually vigorous throughout ninety-eight very full years of life. At last count, he had over forty acknowledged sons living in the United States, not to mention the uncounted scores left behind on the mainland and still living in Taiwan.

The man is a legend in Taiwan, but his story is by no means unusual in the context of Taoist traditions. Though he used tonic herbs most of his life, in interviews he always attributed his health and vitality to

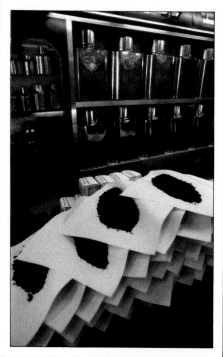

rigorous regimens of exercise, careful diet, and proper personal habits. True enough: tonic herbs alone cannot guarantee health and longevity. But equally true is the fact that without the tonic medicine-wines he imbibed each night before retiring, he could never have practised and benefited from the Way of Yin and Yang and his other healthy Taoist regimens to the advanced age of 98.

Animal-derived medications are prominent among the tonics. Such exotic items as rhinocerous horn, stag horn, the dried genitalia of male sea-lions and seals, the tails of red-spotted lizards, dried sea-horses, gum of tortoise shell and wild donkey hide are all tonics. The reason for their potency is simple: these items contain elements which promote the production of vital-essence. Many of them, such as dried male genitalia and horns, actually contain high concentrations of male hormones because they are the distinguishing male characteristics of the species, and these develop only in the presence of male hormones. Animal-derived tonics are also rich in vital protein substances such as albumins, gelatins, and amino acids. In addition, they contain enzymes, minerals, and trace elements. They have natural affinity for the kidneys and related glands and have a general stimulating effect on the body's vital primordial energies.

Plant-derived items still comprise the majority of tonic herbs. They are considered safer and gentler in action than animal products, and they form the bulk of most tonic prescriptions. Among the most effective tonic herbs are Chinese wolfberry, *Astragalus membranaceus*, *Selincum monnieri*, *Ligustrum japonicum*, red Korean ginseng, and of course the potent Horny Goat Weed. A favoured method of preparing Spring-Wine is to first steep a batch of Horny Goat Weed in the liquor for three to six months, then remove the depleted herb, add all the rest of the tonic ingredients, and steep it for another half year or so before use. When this type of Spring-Wine is imbibed, the Horny Goat Weed first clears the path by dilating all the blood vessels: this permits maximum circulation and distribution of all the other ingredients carried in the wine. Two vital discoveries revealed the connections among sex, longevity, and tonics: Vital-essence (semen and hormones) which promotes vitality and retards aging; and vital-essence which can be nurtured with certain herbs found in nature and preserved by practising the Way of Yin and Yang. A few herbal recipes for Spring-Wine, including the one used by Yang Sen, are given in Chapter Six.

EXTERNAL APPLICATIONS OF CHINESE THERAPY

No system of medicine puts greater emphasis on external forms of therapy than traditional Chinese medicine. Internal and external treatments go hand in hand, regardless of the type of ailment, and few cases are treated without using some form of both methods.

Chinese techniques of external therapy include acupuncture, acupressure, massage, moxibustion, suction cups, blood-letting, skin-scraping, and a wide range of herbal poultices, compresses, and ointments. For internal diseases, the sites chosen for external therapy are vital points and meridians associated with the diseased organ. In case of external ailments or injuries, external therapy is applied directly to the affected areas.

There are eight basic methods of external therapy in Chinese medicine:

ACUPUNCTURE: This form has already been mentioned briefly. The treatment involves insertion of very thin steel needles into vital-energy points along the meridians. Over 800 such points have been identified, although only about 50 are commonly used. Stimulation of the point is achieved by rotating the needles until a tight, twisting sensation is felt at the point by the patient. Every point has specific therapeutic effects on the related organ, specific effects on the body areas covered by the meridian, and a general effect on the body's vital-energy through the meridian complex. Acupuncture can therefore be used to cure diseases of the internal organs as well as to relieve painful symptoms in bones, muscles, joints, and skin. Acupuncture and internal herbal prescriptions are commonly used together.

ACUPRESSURE: Acupressure utilises the same principles and points as acupuncture, but sharp finger pressure rather than needles is used to effect stimulation. Acupressure is often used to simultaneously stimulate two points (one with each hand) while the part of the body in between is twisted and stretched to effect maximum energy flow between the points. Acupressure and massage are usually combined in therapy.

SKIN-SCRAPE: This technique is used for heat-stroke, fever, colds, headache, colic, painful joints, and indigestion. A blunt Chinese soup spoon or a blunt coin is dipped in wine or salt-water and scraped over the patient's skin surface in regular strokes with pressure applied. Another version is to pinch a piece of skin tightly between the big knuckles of the index and middle fingers, pull back sharply, and let it snap back. Both methods are performed rapidly and continuously until bright red stripes appear on the skin. Common sites for skin-scrape therapy are the back of the neck, both sides of the neck, both sides of the Adam's apple, the bridge of the nose, the space between the eyebrows, the upper chest, and along both sides of the spine. This technique relieves symptoms of "hot" and "full" ailments by drawing excess heat and energy to the scraped area, releasing it. It is usually used in combination with cooling yin herbal prescriptions.

BLOOD-LETTING: A sharp triangular needle is used to prick open the site of injury (for external disease) or a vital acupuncture point (for internal disease). A small amount of blood is released. Blood-letting is commonly used for heat stroke, fever, colic, vomiting and diarrhoea, abscesses and swelling, strokes, and traumatic injuries. After the site has been selected, it is routinely sterilised and the skin sharply pricked. The release of blood induces excess "evil-*qi*" and excess heat-energy to escape.

SUCTION CUPS: Suction cups are used against wind-chills, damp-

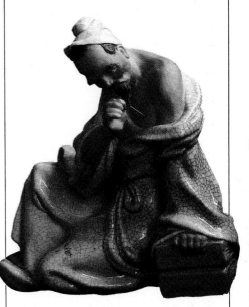

excess, and such common problems as arthritis, rheumatism, abdominal pain, bruises, and abscesses. The cups are made of bamboo or glass and vary in size from a shot-glass to a highball-glass. A piece of cotton held in forceps is dipped in alcohol and ignited. The cup is held mouth-down near the patient and the inside briefly flamed with the burning cotton wad. This reduces air-pressure inside the cup. The cup is then immediately pressed tightly against the site of treatment, to which it adheres

---

OPPOSITE Herbal prescriptions (top) and tea (bottom) are sorted and weighed, ready for sale. ABOVE Ceramic figure of Hua Tuo, claimed to be the "father" of anaesthesia.

firmly by suction. After fifteen to twenty minutes, the cup is released by pressure down on the skin around it and allowing air to enter and equalise the air-pressure. It will leave a bright red circle on the skin, and the treated surface will be beaded with droplets of moisture and, in severe cases, blood. This method literally sucks out excess moisture, chills, dampness, and leaked blood from the areas treated.

MASSAGE (*Tui Na*): Chinese massage techniques are simple and effective. Massage clears the meridians of blockages, stimulates circulation of

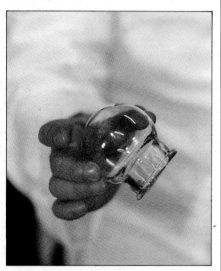

blood and energy, loosens stiff joints and muscles, and raises vitality and resistances to disease. It is most commonly used in cases of acute back strain, sprained joints, pulled muscles and tendons, rheumatism and arthritis, nerve paralysis, prolapse of internal organs, sciatica, and similar ailments. There are many massage techniques, but the most common and effective focus on the nerve centres and meridians that run from the base of the neck down to the heels, especially along either side of the spinal column. The ball of the thumb is used to alternately push hard then rub lightly along and around the site of massage. This method simultaneously stimulates the internal organs connected to the meridians and nerves while it tones up the muscles, tendons and ligaments through which the nerves and meridians run. Massage therapy is often followed up with herbal poultices and pills.

MOXIBUSTION: This therapeutic method employs a burning moxa wick placed directly over the skin at vital points. "Moxa" is derived from Japanese and means "burning herb". It is a soft, downy material obtained from a variety of herbs, which is rolled tightly in rice paper to form tubes about the size of a large cigar. One end is ignited until it glows evenly, then it is held about an inch from the skin over a vital point and rotated slowly. Its healing effects radiate directly through the skin to influence the meridian below. The most common herb used for moxibustion is Chinese wormwood, *Arte-*

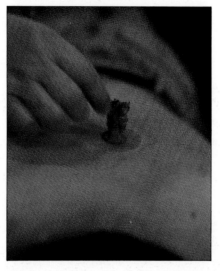

misia vulgaris. It is used for a wide variety of ailments, including mumps, chronic nose-bleeds, vaginal bleeding, arthritis and rheumatism, pulled nerves, numbness in muscles, and others.

HERBAL POULTICES: Herbal poultices employ many of the same ingredients used for internal herbal prescriptions. The herbs are first ground to a very fine powder and mixed dry for storage. Just before use, some powder is mixed with a little water until the texture of peanut-butter is achieved. This is spread thickly over a piece of cloth or wax-paper, stuck tightly over the injured area, and taped in place for eight to twelve hours. The combination of moisture and body heat activates the herbal mix, which draws out excess "evil-*qi*" and radiates in healing vapours. Herbal poultices are used for arthritic and rheumatic conditions, strained backs, sprained joints and tendons,

blocked meridians, nervous disorders, bruising, swelling, and abscesses. They are usually applied after massage or acupressure therapy. Sometimes several of the major ingredients of the poultice will also appear in an internal prescription to be taken during the course of treatment.

The external therapeutic techniques described above can all be combined with internal herbal treatments, and they all follow the theoretical guidelines of yin-yang and the Five Elements. As usual, syncretism—not specialisation—is the key. Just as the Chinese often burn

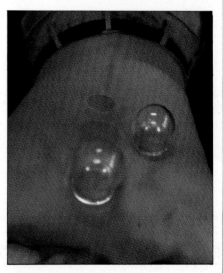

insense and make offerings simultaneously to several gods of different religious traditions—just to make sure they're covered by all—so Chinese doctors often employ two or three different therapeutic methods against the same ailment, just to make sure the treatment hits the mark.

FOOD, SEX, AND LONGEVITY

"Food and sex are natural," admitted the great sage Confucius over 2,000 years ago. Civilised as he was, even Confucius could not deny the fundamental nature of these two functions.

Food and sex are the only two indispensable requirements for the

Suction cups and moxibustion (ABOVE and RIGHT) are used in the treatment of rheumatism and muscular pain — the cups drawing out "dampness" and leaked blood, and the moxibustion heat radiating down into vital meridiens.

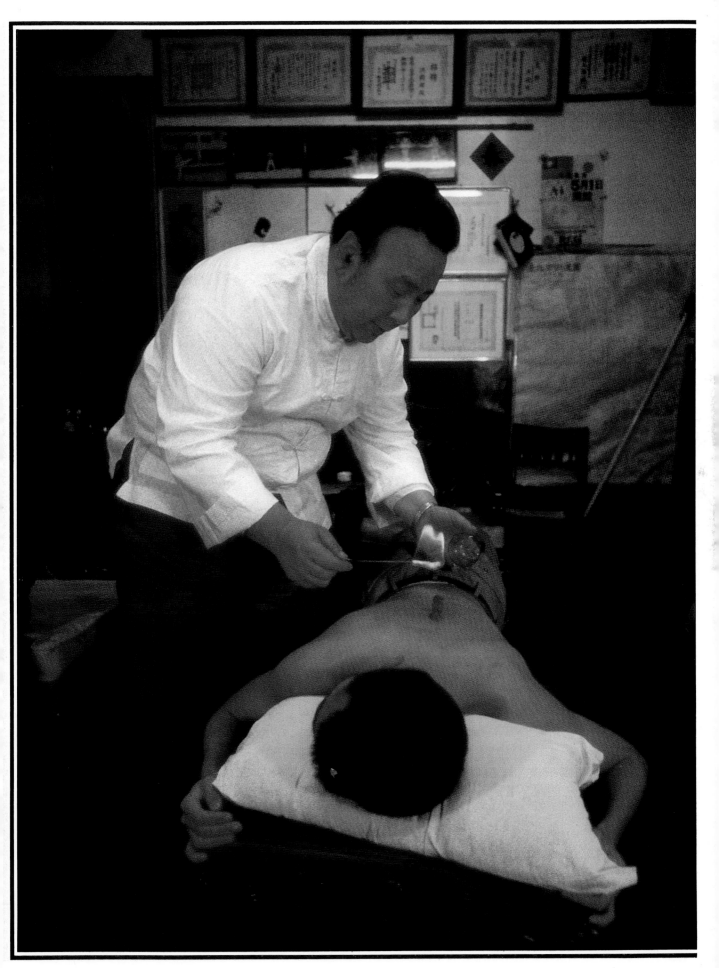

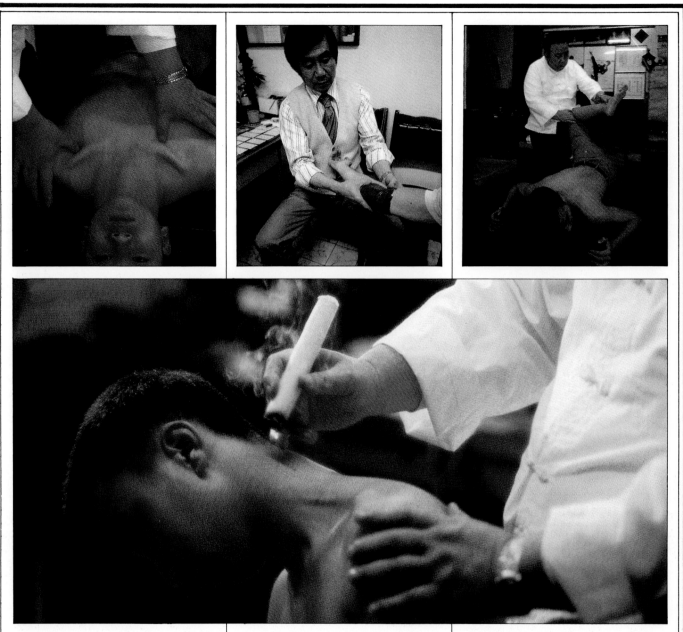

survival and propagation of the species. All else is superfluous. They are the strongest natural instincts and the most basic functions we have. As such, food and sex are also the most fundamental indicators of health and disease and the best means of attaining longevity.

Food, above all, is the constant cure and forms the foundation of Chinese preventive medicine. If proper dietary habits are cultivated, even when disease does strike, its effects are far less debilitating, and recovery is quick. In China, food is medicine.

Chinese herbal medicine is so closely tied to food that the two are inseparable. Some foods act as specific catalysts for certain herbal medications, while other foods completely neutralise them. Such foods are either recommended or prohibited during treatment with Chinese herbs. Foods are categorised according to the same classifications used to distinguish herbs: Four Energies (hot, warm, cold, cool); Five Flavours (hot, sweet, sour, bitter, salty); yin and yang; tonic-sedative; etc. Herbal prescriptions are sometimes mixed right into common foods, while others must be taken on an empty stomach. Much that appears on the spice shelf in Western kitchens is commonly used in Chinese herbal medicine. In China, the realms of the kitchen and the clinic overlap, and indeed most herbal prescriptions are prepared for consumption in the kitchen. Chinese physicians try to follow Sun Simiao's ancient dictum: first try food; resort to medication only when food fails to effect a cure. Food is the first line of defense in traditional Chinese medicine.

The principles involved in food therapy are identical to those of herbal therapy. After consuming a meal rich in "hot" food items, such as lamb, ginger, peanuts, chilis, etc., you can prevent the symptoms of internal "heat-excess" simply by taking a few "cool" foods for desert, such as fresh oranges or limes, watermelon (the coolest of all), papaya, and so forth. Chinese chefs have always been familiar with the pharmaceutical nature of the foods they cook with, and therefore the average Chinese banquet strikes a fine balance not only in flavour, aroma, texture, and colour, but also in the energies and essences they impart to the body upon digestion. After the banquet, you sometimes "feel hungry an hour later" not because of insufficient quantity but because of superior quality and balance. Good Chinese food mixes well in the stomach, digests easily, and is distributed rapidly throughout the system.

A regulated, healthy sexual life is the other side of the coin of longevity. In *Precious Recipes* Sun Simiao tells us:

A man can live a healthy and long life if he carries out an emission frequency of two times monthly or twenty-four times yearly. If at the same time he also pays attention to wholesome food and exercises, he may attain longevity.

Dr. Sun lived to the age of 101 by following his own advice. His personal schedule of emission was once every hundred coitions, though he considered this too strict a regimen for the average man. In another seventh-century treatise called *Longevity Principles*, Master Liu Ching gives us his version of regulated sex for men:

In Spring, a man can permit himself to ejaculate once in three days. In Summer and Autumn, twice a month. During cold Winter, one should save semen and not ejaculate at all. The way of Heaven is to accumulate Yang-essence during Winter. A man will attain longevity if he follows this yardstick. One ejaculation in cold Winter is one hundred times more harmful than in Springtime.

One therapeutic effect of Spring-Wine is to tonify and strengthen the tissue of the ureter and seminal-vessels so that retention techniques can be successfully employed. Not only have these Taoist practices been used effectively to maintain health and prolong life by countless generations of Chinese adepts, their underlying medical principles have also been confirmed by recent scientific research in the West.

In a study conducted in 1974 at the Max Planck Institute of Psychiatry in Munich, researchers discovered a significant increase in testosterone levels in the blood of 75 percent of men who were shown a mildly erotic film. Imagine how much more effective real sexual activity is in securing high hormone levels in the blood! German scientists subsequently discovered that men with high hormone levels, high sperm count, and dense semen have unusually high resistance to some diseases and absolute immunity to others! This was heralded as a "great new discovery" in the international press.

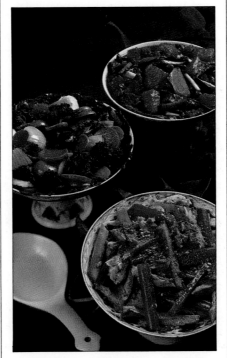

Chinese physicians, however, have always maintained that insufficient vital-hormone production— "empty kidney-glands", results in low resistance to disease and a short life-span. The herbal tonics they prescribe for this condition stimulate hormone production, raise sperm count, and thicken the semen. The purpose of this therapy is not aphrodisiac—although that is sometimes a side-effect in healthy persons—but medical: it is meant to increase vitality, strengthen resistance, and promote longevity. Taoist techniques of retaining semen to preserve the vital-essence may be viewed as the complementary form of external therapy to internal herbal tonics.

Longevity has always been the most prized and respected achievement among the Chinese people. Their idea of longevity, however, does not envision years spent in wheelchairs and sanatoria, sexual impotence, inability to eat and digest properly, nervous disorders, senility, and other common attendant evils of old age in the West. The Chinese expect to live out their years in health and vitality, remaining fully active and alert to the end. Chinese herbal medicine, especially of the tonic variety, is thus employed most often by people moving from middle into old age, when the body begins to degenerate at a faster rate, and food and sex unaided are no longer enough to effectively retard the aging process.

Herbal medicines promote longevity both by improving the tone of muscles, organs, and other tissues and by stimulating their natural functions, so that as the body ages it can continue to derive maximum benefits from food, sex, exercise, breathing, and other regimens. Tonifying the body with expensive herbal concoctions only to ruin it with poor food, a reckless sex life, and bad habits is obviously going to be self-defeating. On the other hand, herbs can double and even triple the benefits the body derives from the good food, regulated sex, and healthy habits. This is especially true as one gets older. Chinese herbal preparations act as the great balancers of the body, the traffic directors of the complex cross-currents of vital-energies and cosmic forces which constantly course through our bodies. They promote health and longevity but do not guarantee them. This is a most important point to remember. Herbs can only keep the body and its many functional parts well balanced and in good working order: the rest is up to you.

OPPOSITE In the treatment of rheumatism, sciatica, strain and nerve paralysis, massage is used along with herbal poultices and moxibustion. ABOVE Diet is enlisted too into the vast armoury of the herbal physician.

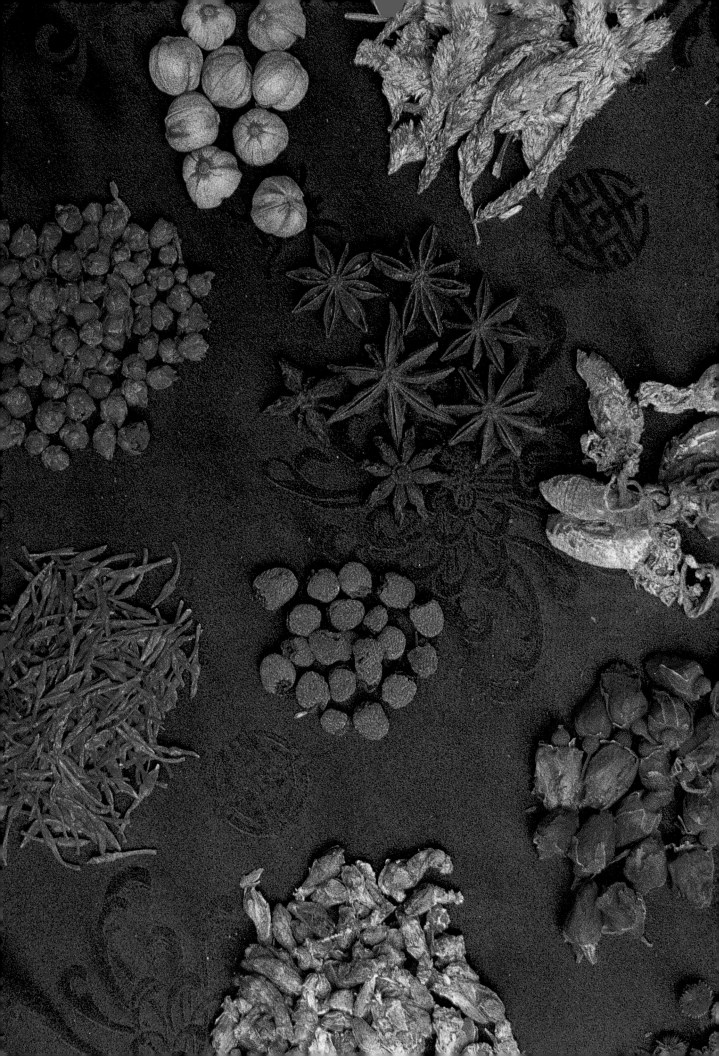

Chapter V

The Perennial Cornucopia

Chinese Herbal Medicine Today

hinese herbal medicine still relies upon the vast domains of nature, which constantly replenish themselves despite the deprecations of man. As long as there are sunshine and rain, trees and flowers, animals and fish, earth and sea, there will always be sources of herbal medicine. Nature hasn't changed much since the dawn of Chinese herbal arts, over 5,000 years ago. Neither have the underlying theories and basic techniques of traditional Chinese medicine, which are patterned precisely after nature. However, new herbs, new prescriptions, new applications, and new insights based on the age-old knowledge are

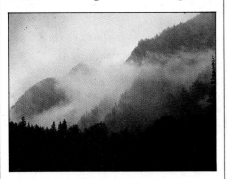

being developed every day by contemporary practitioners of the ancient art of Chinese healing. In this chapter, we first take a brief look at the sources of Chinese herbs today, how they are gathered, dried, and stored, and where they are sold. Then we will cover some recent modern developments in the field and look in on two contemporary Chinese physicians—a Taoist and a Confucianist—who still practice the ancient art in the modern world.

GROWING, GATHERING, DRYING, AND STORING THE HERBS

The best Chinese herbs grow naturally in China. Ever since the earliest beginnings, the craggy mountains and deep valleys of Sichuan have provided the richest sources of potent wild herbs, those which depend on

Part of the "vast domains of nature" (RIGHT & OPPOSITE) that contribute to the immense pharmacopoeia of traditional Chinese medicine.

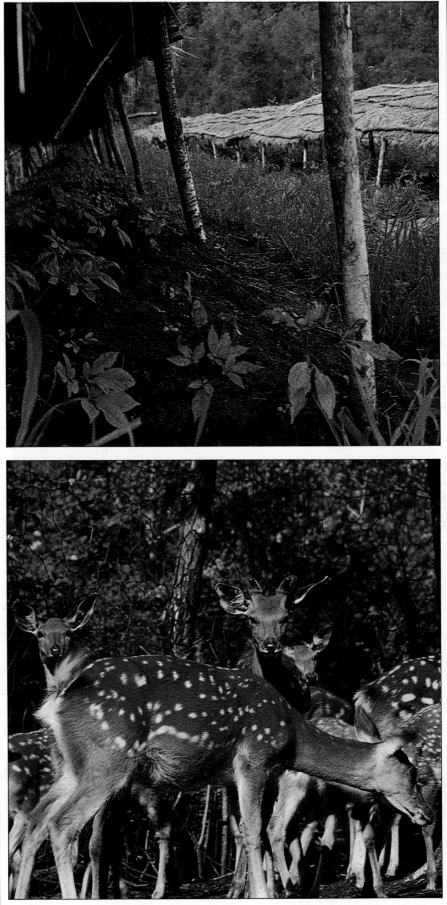

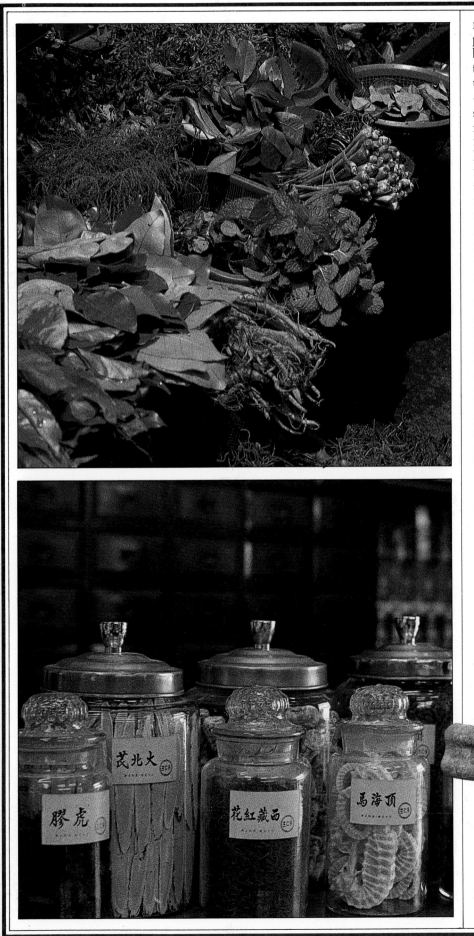

nature, not man, for growth and propagation. Many of these cannot be cultivated: they must be sought in their wild, natural surroundings. The unique conditions of geography and climate which prevail in Sichuan seem to suit the requirements of many of the most useful wild herbs. Some plants thrive in extremely harsh conditions, and this environmental adversity seems to be the source of their potency. Some of the more potent herbs, such as ginseng root, leave the soil in which they are found totally depleted, and nothing else will grow in the same spot for many years after the herb is gathered.

The other southern provinces, such as Yunnan, Guizhou, Guangxi, and Guangdong, also abound with the natural flora and fauna which provide the raw materials of the *ben cao*. Cultivated herbs—those which depend on artificial seed selection, grafting, fertilisation, irrigation, and other human help—grow well in the temperate lush regions of south China. The cultivation of medicinal plants is a major agricultural industry in this region of China.

Northern China is home to many of the potent tonic plants, such as ginseng, *Astragalus membranaceus*, and *Lycium chinense*. It is also in the north where the famous spotted deer is found: everything from the velvet and horns to the blood and bile of the spotted deer is used in Chinese medicine. Today, spotted deer are raised on large ranches in Manchuria and other northern provinces to meet the great demand for one of the most potent and popular tonics—spotted deer horn. The horns are cut from the live deer—a painful process for the animal—so that the same herd can be used to produce the precious material year after year. When the deer get too old to regenerate new horns, the entire animal is used for its many medicinally useful parts.

New sources of medicinal ingredients which can be used in Chinese herbal medicine are constantly being sought. Southeast Asia provides a number of the plants and animals required. Even North America exports an herbal item to the Far East called "American Gingseng." It is a different species of ginseng which grows wild in North America; it is quite potent, and fetches a good price on the Asian herb market. Northern states of America such as Minnesota and North Dakota have recently begun exporting deer horn to the Far East as well.

Mineral and animal derived medicines from non-Chinese sources are generally more acceptable than plants which are far more specific and sensitive to the unique conditions of soil and weather which prevail in China. The essential energies, flavour, and effects of the myriad herbs used in Chinese medicine were determined from the varieties native to China. Varieties of the same plants which grow elsewhere can have very different pharmaceutical properties, and it takes centuries to fully determine their natural affinities and pharmacodynamic effects. Fortunately for overseas Chinese communities, modern transportation has made it possible for the genuine articles to be shipped from China.

The parts of the plant used for medicinal purposes differ in each variety of herb. In some plants, only the roots are medically useful; in others, only the stems, flowers, seeds or leaves are used. There are also plants which are used whole and ones whose every part is used for widely different purposes. For example, the roots and stems of the herb *ma huang* (*Ephedra sinica*) contain the bronchial asthma preventive, ephedrine, but the joints have a completely opposite action and are used for totally different purposes. Since different parts of plants mature and become medically active at different times of the year, it is important to gather the medicinal parts of each variety at just the right time.

Roots and rhizomes, which grow below ground, are most potent in late autumn and early spring, when the bulk of plant nutrients are stored in them. Barks are collected between February and May, when their moisture content is highest. Most leaves are gathered just before the flowers begin to bloom, although some varieties may be collected in the autumn, when they begin to drop.

When gathering medicinal flowers, timing is even more important because the flowering season for most plants is generally quite short. Flowers

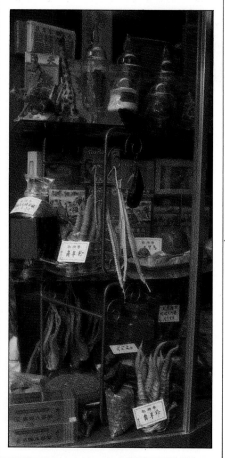

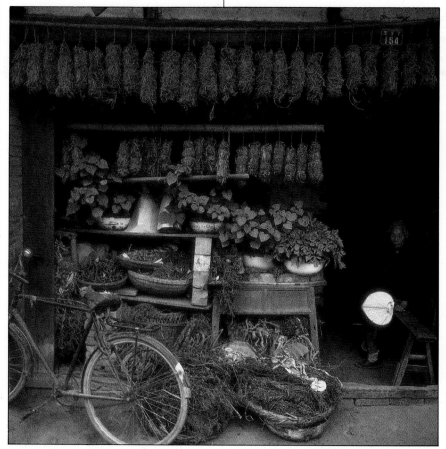

are gathered between March and May and during July and August, depending on when they begin to bloom. They should be picked in bud or after just having burst into bloom. They must be sun-dried immediately.

Fruits used in herbal medicine are usually picked upon ripening. However, there are a few varieties, such as *wu mei* ("black-plums," *Prunus mume*), which are used unripened, and they should be picked earlier. Seeds used in herbal medicine are also collected after they have completely matured. Some are gathered directly from the ground, while others are collected from the ripe, withered fruit before it splits apart.

After the herbs have been gathered, they must be properly processed for maximum drug efficacy. The first step is to sort the herbs. On a typical day of herb gathering, the picker's basket will contain a variety of plants and plant parts, depending on which plants and parts are in season and mature that day. Dirt, impurities, and non-medicinal parts are first removed from all the plants. Then the plants and parts with different uses are separated.

After sorting, the plants should be washed well to remove remaining dirt and dust. Before washing, flowers must be removed and dried separately. A few plants, such as plantain and green bristlegrass, should not be washed at all.

When the plants have been gathered, sorted, and washed, they are ready for drying. Most herbs are dried in direct sunshine, which insures best storage. During the rainy season or on cloudy days, the herbs may be dried indoors around a fire. Aromatics such as mint are dried in well-ventilated shade. Animal parts must first be steamed to kill parasites, eggs, and germs before drying.

When they are thoroughly dry, the plants are sliced into convenient sizes and shapes for storage. Thick roots, rhizomes, and woody vines are cut into thin slices. Barks and leaves are shaved into long, fine strips. Whole plants are divided into sections. Flowers and seeds are stored and shipped whole. After cutting and sectioning, different items should immediately be labeled to prevent mis-identification and misuse

of the drugs. When they get to the herbal shop, they are stored in wooden drawers, ceramic vessels, and glass bottles, always in a cool, dry, well-ventilated place. The stored herbs should be inspected regularly for mildew, bugs, oil loss, and other damage. They are sun-aired frequently, especially during the damp rainy season, to prevent such damage.

In gathering wild herbs, it is vital to avoid over-picking an area and to take the long-range view in protecting these precious resources. A planned schedule of collection should be followed, gathering only enough for current needs and considering future requirements. If possible, parts should be picked in such a way that the entire plant does not perish. Roots should be left in the soil whenever possible. If roots are the parts to be collected, the main tap root should be left intact. When gathering leaves, a single plant should never be stripped clean, or it will die. The same applies to barks.

Comprehensive, systematic utilisation of both wild and cultivated herbs is essential to ensure adequate

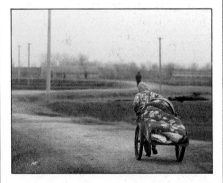

supplies of vital ingredients. Whenever wasteland or forests are cleared for agricultural use, for example, a thorough inspection of the areas to be cleared should first be made and all medically-useful plants gathered. No plant materials should be discarded or burned until their potential medical uses have been determined. Medicinal plants which adapt well to cultivation should be planted wherever possible on land reclaimed

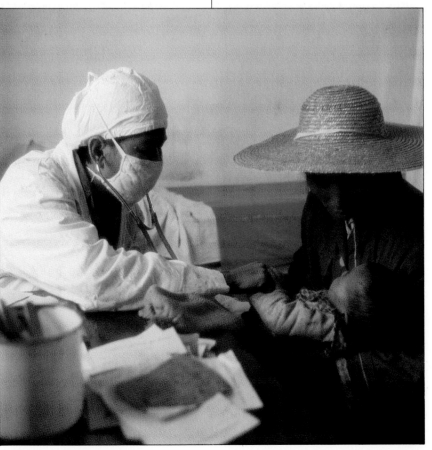

OPPOSITE With herbal medicines, as with their everyday foods, the Chinese prefer to see exactly what they're buying. LEFT "Barefoot" doctor and patient in post-revolutionary China. ABOVE "Barefoot" rural ambulance.

from the wild, on the banks of streams and ponds, on the edges of paddy-fields, and on road-sides. Proper planning and planting ensure sufficient supplies of herbs for normal needs as well as back-up reserves for sudden emergencies.

THE HERBAL TRADE

Today, Chinese herbs are available in Chinese herb shops in many parts of the world, thanks to the demands of the far-flung overseas Chinese communities. Most large cities, East or West, with a Chinese community

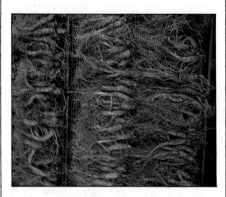

and a few Chinese restaurants have at least one well-stocked Chinese herb shop.

The Chinese herbal trade centres around Hong Kong, China's main commercial outlet to the world for close to 150 years. After the herbs have been gathered and processed in China, they are carefully inspected for quality; only the best are offered for sale on the international market. Top quality herbs fetch high prices and for some really rare, exotic but potent tonics the prices may attract only the richest of overseas Chinese tycoons but the total sum contributes significantly to China's foreign exchange reserves.

The herbs are sold retail at the herb counters of special China-product emporiums in Hong Kong, as well as at the hundreds of private little herb shops which flourish there. Wholesalers in Hong Kong supply both the local retailers and the international market. The further away from Hong Kong you go, the more expensive the drugs become. Hong Kong is a Mecca for Chinese herbal enthusiasts because everything is available, the quality is the best, and

the prices are more reasonable.

Is US$10,000 a reasonable price to pay for a single ounce of an exotic variety of ginseng root? Would you pay US$250 for a tiny shrivelled black wad, purported to be the dried testicle of a rare breed of deer? In Hong Kong, these are the sort of prices asked and fetched, demonstrating that certain people are willing to pay that much to obtain them. The reason they are willing to pay so much is because a few extra years, months, or even weeks of healthy life are more precious to the Chinese than "all the tea in China." Such items are, of course, the Cadillacs of Chinese herbs, and only wealthy individuals can afford them. But there are items on the Chinese herbalist's shelves to suit every budget and every need, and indeed many of the best drugs are quite common and inexpensive. Chinese herbal prescriptions are, more often than not, less expensive than their chemical Western counterparts and thus more generally available to the common people. Men and women, young and old, rich and poor alike, almost all Chinese the world over resort to herbal remedies at least sometimes during their life.

Occasionally the most popular and potent herbal medicines are subject to the fluctuations of supply and demand. For example, *Yunnan bai yao*, the healing white powder made from "mountain varnish," is today in ample supply at any medicine counter in Hong Kong for less than US$2.00 a vial. Only a few years ago, however, during the height of the Vietnam War, it was usually impossible to find at any price. The entire supply was being sent to the North Vietnamese Army, where the precious powder became a part of every soldier's field kit. Recall that the other name for this herb is "gold-no-trade." The Chinese sometimes have to make careful choices between commercial and benevolent motives when distributing limited supplies of healing herbs.

Taiwan, today one of the wealthiest, also one of the most traditional Chinese communities in the world, has the greatest demand for high-quality Chinese herbs. However, due to the long-standing hostility between Taipei and Beijing, formal trade

between the two cousins is banned. While the government in Taiwan authorises certain firms in Hong Kong to purchase limited amounts of vital mainland herbs for transshipment to Taiwan, this legal supply comes nowhere close to meeting actual demands, especially for the more exotic tonics. Furthermore, import duties are astronomical, driving prices sky-high. Consequently, a bustling illegal trade across the Taiwan Straits brings close to US$10 million worth of precious Chinese herbs to Taiwan each year. It is significant that whenever Taiwanese fishing boats are caught smuggling contraband between Taiwan and the China coast, the items brought back to Taiwan are usually priceless antiques, gold bars, and Chinese herbs. Even politics cannot stand between the Chinese people and their beloved herbal remedies.

MODERN DEVELOPMENTS

Despite its well established theories and techniques, Chinese herbal medicine continues to develop dynamically in the modern world. It is unfortunate that the orthodox medical establishment in the West remains leery of Chinese medical theories and practises, for the Chinese system holds profound insights and effective remedies from which the whole world should benefit.

One modern development already alluded to is the production of patent herbal medicines refined from extracts of the crude herbs. These medications cannot be relied upon for acute or serious ailments. In such cases, specific herbal prescriptions based on differential diagnosis must be obtained from qualified Chinese doctors. For chronic ailments and long-standing weaknesses, however, the patent herbal potions are quite effective. They contain the essential ingredients required for gradual and constant tonification of the internal organs. Such modern Chinese medicines as Royal Jelly Capsules, Deer-Testicle Pills, Great Tonic Pills, Deer Horn Extract, Essence of Ginseng, and many others are all mild but effective tonics when used regularly over an extended period of time.

Another development made possible by modern technology is extracting and refining the active ingredients of the crude herbs until a very concentrated, pure essence is obtained. This herbal essence is injected directly into vital energy points along the major meridians. Due to the herb's natural affinity for a specific organ, the herbal essence has an immediate effect on that organ's meridian when injected directly into one of its vital points. The effect is then transmitted to the organ through the meridian network. This is a more recent development in Chinese herbal medicine and holds much promise. It is interesting to note that this modern application of the ancient art has been made possible by modern Western technology.

Perhaps the most promising contemporary development in the ancient field of Chinese herbal medicine is the discovery of an herb which can be safely used for birth control. Dr. Y. C. Kong, biochemist and master Chinese herbalist at The Chinese University of Hong Kong, is currently heading a multi-million dollar research project sponsored by the World Health Organisation to develop a safe, effective herbal contraceptive. He has already discovered the plant which he thinks will help control the world's exploding population. "We are convinced the plant can be used as an effective means of preventing gestation," he states. Furthermore, the herb grows naturally and in abundance throughout most of the world's tropical and subtropical zones. "Women in most developing countries will be able to gather or grow it and make a tea out of it." The herbal contraceptive works "the morning after" and apparently has no ill side effects. Dr. Kong has been besieged by offers from pharmaceutical companies to sell his

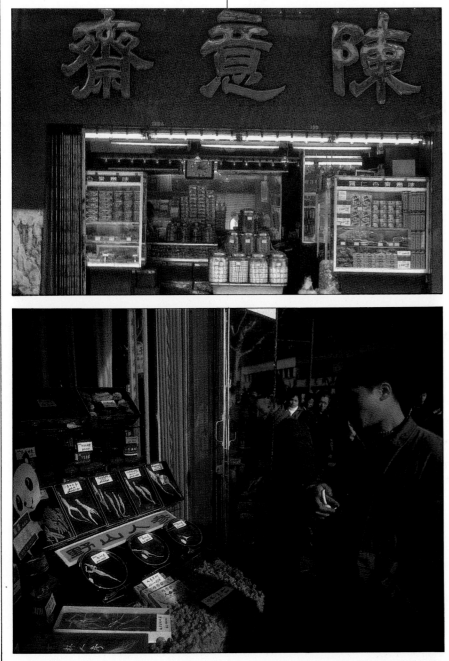

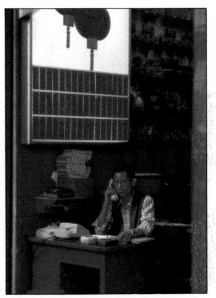

secret for this potential panacea for the world's population problem, but he remains adamant in his insistence that the public interest be served first. In about two years, when research on the plant's long-term effects and toxicity are complete, he will turn the results over to the World Health Organisation to utilize as they see fit.

In the Far East, the process of melding traditional Chinese and modern Western approaches to medical care is already well under way. The resulting hybrid system is generally referred to as the "New

OPPOSITE Wild ginseng, one of the most popular tonics in East Asia. LEFT Two contrasting herbal medicine stores in China. ABOVE Characters list the various herbs and potions available for sale.

Medicine." New Medicine relies heavily on such aspects of modern Western technology as integrated scientific laboratories, X-ray, chemical analysis, microscopic biochemistry, refining and purifying techniques, electronics, optics, and others. But when it comes to the fundamental theories of disease and the practical applications of therapy, the Chinese system is generally followed.

In China today, Chinese and Western medical approaches are practised side by side. The official Chinese paramedical manual, called *A Barefoot Doctor's Manual* (see bibliography), gives both alternative and combined Chinese and Western treatments for every type of disease discussed. At an agricultural commune's clinic in Anhui Province, a Western journalist asked the head physician whether he relies more on Chinese or Western methods in the treatment of disease. "Both," the doctor answered without hesitation. But how does the physician know when to apply which method, the journalist wanted to know. "By experience," was the doctor's confident and characteristically Chinese response.

The Chinese have always been open to new experience and experimentation in the field of medicine, which is why their medical system has always been the most compre-

hensive, effective, and flexible in the world. It remains so today. Perhaps it is fitting that more work is being done in the East on the New Medicine. Grafting scientific investigative disciplines onto an empirical system may be less of a leap in perception than moving from scientific disciplines to embrace the less quantifiable "Wisdom of the East."

MODERN PRACTITIONERS OF THE ANCIENT ART

Just as Chinese herbal shops and herbal remedies have changed little since the Song and Ming dynasties, Chinese physicians have also continued to practise their ancient healing arts according to the traditions and standards established by their forefathers in the field. Such great Chinese physicians as Hua Tuo, Sun Simiao, and Li Shizhen of the late Han, early Tang and Ming dynasties respectively, would have felt very much at home in the clinics of some modern-day practitioners. Contemporary Chinese doctors have found little use for most of the therapeutic chemicals and equipment found in typical Western clinics. They do, however, combine some basic Western diagnostic techniques, such as X-rays, blood-pressure, blood and urine analysis, etc., with their own traditional diagnostic methods.

One of our examples of contemporary Chinese physician, of the Confucian tradition in Chinese medicine, is Dr. Huang Powen, who has conducted a small clinic in Taipei for the past twenty-five years. He is master of the traditional Chinese massage method called "push-and-rub," *tui na*, which he combines in therapy with acupuncture, herbal poultices, and internal herbal prescriptions. His patients come from all walks of life—high government officals, house-wives, American businessmen, Chinese secretaries, Arabian oil-sheiks and local cab-drivers. The walls of his clinic are covered with framed letters from his patients, expressions of effusive praise and heartfelt gratitude.

Like the great Tang physician Sun Simiao, Dr. Huang has refused many lucrative offers to become personal

private physician to ailing men of great wealth and power. He prefers, instead, to remain in his humble clinic and fulfill his sacred obligations to his many patients. One, a wealthy Lebanese tycoon who suffers from a painful chronic sciatic condition, offered to pay his roundtrip fare first-class between Taipei and Beirut, plus a fantastic fee, to treat him at his home in Beirut for a month! Citing the many patients who rely daily on his "benevolent heart, benevolent art," the benevolent doctor politely declined. So, the tycoon flew to Taipei and Dr. Huang treated him in his suite at the Hilton Hotel after closing up his clinic at night.

Huang Powen is a native Taiwanese whose family has been practising *tui na* massage, acupuncture, and herbal medicine for several generations. Asked what the main sources of his profound knowledge and exceptional skills were, he replied, "My family and my own experience." He holds all the necessary government licenses to practise Chinese medicine but insists that these are mere formalities. Difficult as the Chinese medical examinations are, passing them only proves that one has mastered the theories and memorised the mass of medical and herbal terminology required to practise the art. Skill, insight, clinical experience, special

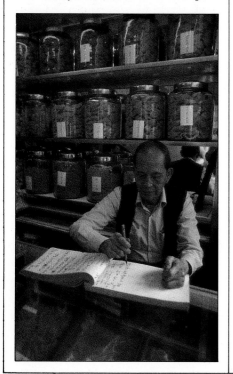

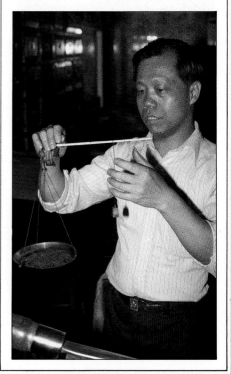

techniques passed from master to apprentice, and a refined personal touch combine to elevate an ordinary doctor to an exceptional one.

Dr. Huang recommends internal herbal prescriptions and properly balanced diets as complementary supplements to his external therapies of *tui na* massage and herbal poultices. It is not uncommon for Chinese doctors to develop remedies based on their own clinical experience and interest. Dr. Huang is certainly no exception to this practice; the herbal poultice he applies after massage evolved in this way and contains 16 herbal ingredients. It is highly effective in cases of rheumatism and arthritis, strained backs and sprained joints, sciatica and other nerve disorders, twisted tendons and pulled muscles, energy and blood stagnation, bruises and abscesses, windchills, and other related conditions.

An elderly American woman on tour in Taipei was once brought to him for treatment of acute, unbearable pain resulting from a sudden flare-up of a pinched nerve in her spine, which had plagued her for over 20 years. Her Western-prescribed treatment for this condition for the past two decades was a bottle of powerful pain-killers: "take two or three for pain." This time, however, even these did nothing to alleviate her misery. She was prepared to cancel her trip and return to New York on a stretcher under sedation when a Chinese acquaintance insisted that she try Dr. Huang. After her first treatment, she felt so much better that she decided to stay and complete her tour of Taiwan. After her second *tui na* massage and herbal poultice, she burst into grateful tears before the doctor and said, "It's a miracle." She vowed to return to Taipei for further treatment.

More recently, Dr. Huang has developed his own secret prescription of herbal ingredients to be taken internally as an herbal broth for relief of the same conditions he treats with massage and poultice. The internal and external herbal treatments work together to eliminate the painful symptoms and correct the causes of the conditions mentioned above. This potion is so effective that other Chinese doctors suffering from these ailments visit Dr. Huang to obtain relief with his secret elixir.

It is common practice for Chinese physicians to visit other renowned doctors as patients, first of all to seek relief for ailments in which other doctors specialise, and secondly to obtain samples of secret prescriptions in hopes of duplicating them. For example, Dr. Huang, who recently suffered from a stubborn liver inflammation, paid several visits to a Taiwanese doctor whose secret herbal remedy for serious liver ailments was reported to be extremely effective. Liver ailments are particularly difficult to cure completely. "The poisons were quickly driven out of my liver and brought to the surface by this prescription. My skin was mottled, itchy, sticky, and smelly for several weeks during the treatment, and then I was completely cured," he reports. So impressed was Dr. Huang with the quick effective cure that he has begun the long and arduous task of deciphering the prescription's secret formula.

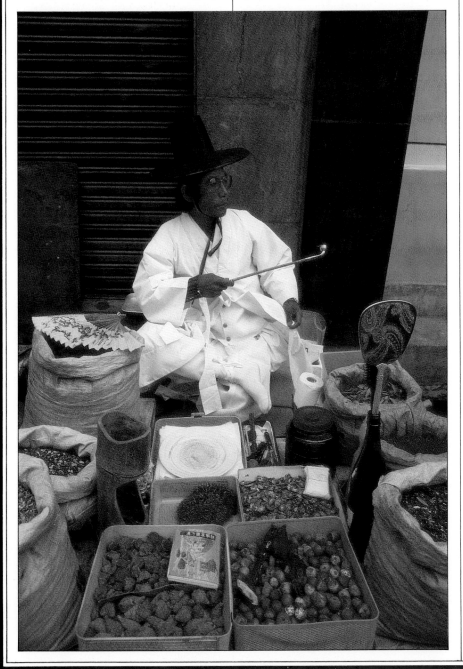

LEFT A travelling Korean physician. In Korea, like China, travelling physicians offer their herbal remedies throughout the country. *Photo: Alain Evrard.* OPPOSITE Weighing herbal ingredients with traditional balance and (for left) entering items in a ledger.

Professional physicians like Dr. Huang maintain the finest traditions of Confucian benevolence and are responsible for making the benefits of China's ancient healing arts directly available to the common people. The average cost of a half-hour massage and/or acupuncture treatment, including an herbal poultice, run at less than half of what it costs just to walk into a private doctor's office in the West and say, "Ahhh." Furthermore, Dr. Huang charges even less to those who cannot afford it and accepts more from those wealthy patients who willingly offer it. He won't be found on the golf-course on week-ends, nor is the doctor ever "out." Dr. Huang lives in a modest apartment directly above his clinic and answers patients' calls any time of day or night. For him, as for his Confucian forerunners, the practice of Chinese medicine is a full-time, lifetime commitment.

On the other side of town lives and practises a Chinese doctor of the Taoist tradition, Dr. Hong Yixiang, our other contemporary example. His philosophic persuasions and life-style are as different from Dr. Huang's as those of Confucius were from Lao Zi, the founding father of Taoism. He practises the syncretic, total approach to health and disease handed down by such great Taoist physicians as Hua Tuo and Sun Simiao. His commitment is more to the art of healing itself than to society at large.

Like Dr. Huang, Dr. Hong favours the external forms of Chinese therapy combined with internal herbal supplements. The theories and methods they employ are drawn from the same ancient canons and herbal pharmacopoeias. Dr. Hong's preferred techniques are acupressure and massage, moxibustion, and suction cups, and he uses them for both internal and external ailments. His clinic is quite similar to Dr. Huang's, and he too lives in an apartment attached to the clinic. But this is where the similarity ends.

In addition to being a qualified, licensed Chinese doctor, Hong Yixiang is also one of the greatest living masters of the Chinese martial arts. He has been practising the medical and martial arts side by side for nearly thirty years at his home in

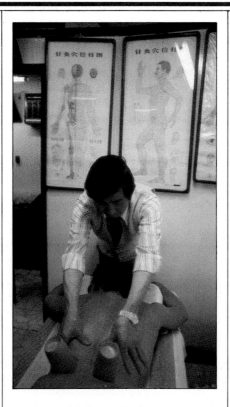

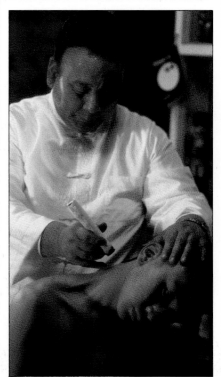

ABOVE Bamboo beakers are sometimes used instead of glass cups for suction treatment, applied along with massage and moxibustion. BELOW Dr Huang Po Wen OPPOSITE Dr Hong Yixiang.

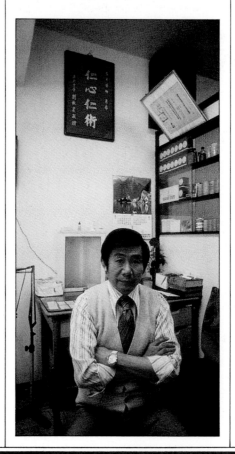

a narrow lane off a small street deep in the west side of Taipei. He draws upon the martial arts for medical therapy, and uses herbal medicine to improve the performance of, and repair injuries sustained by, his kung-fu students in class.

Hong Yixiang follows the "soft" path of traditional Chinese kung-fu, which relies on the internal power of qi rather than external muscular strength. He has combined the three classical soft styles of xing yi, "form of will," ba gua "eight trigrams," and tai ji quan, "ultimate supreme fist" to found his own school of kung-fu called Tang shou dao, "the way of the hands of Tang." In the grand Chinese tradition, his first two mentors were his grandfather and his father. Subsequently, he studied under seventeen famous Chinese masters, each of whom specialised in specific forms and imparted precious secrets to him. His three sons and the handful of students who are lucky enough to find and be accepted by him study Tang shou dao under his tutelage in a small kung-fu studio attached to clinic.

Hong Yixiang defies the image of the kung-fu master commonly held in the West. Neither the handsome, dashing young adventurer like the late Bruce Lee, nor the wizened, white-bearded old man in robes,

Hong Yixiang stands about 5 ft 6 in (1.68 m) tall and weighs well over 200 lb (90.8 kg). His clothing is nondescript, he generally appears unshaven, and he walks with a slow, ambling shuffle. He has the long *Luohan* ear-lobes which Buddhists identify as a sign of high spiritual development. Yet to watch him demonstrate his subtle fighting forms is a stark lesson in contrast and contradiction: he controls his massive bulk with the agility of a cat, his every movement is soft and smooth as water, swift and sudden as lightning, and effortless as the wind. He has mastered control of his *qi* to such a degree that he can concentrate and direct the full bulk of his weight and the full force of his internal power on a single point. Should that point happen to be your heart or lungs or kidney or other vital spot, you would perish instantly. To complete the contrast, when the fist which commands such immense power relaxes and takes up the Chinese brush, it becomes the delicate hand of an accomplished Chinese painter and calligrapher: Hong Yixiang is indeed a man of many talents, an archetype, adept at the ancient Taoist arts.

Qi is the great secret of Chinese medicine as well as Chinese kung-fu. As such, it is the common denominator linking the medical and martial arts. Dr. Hong teaches his students breathing exercise which improve the quality and increase the quantity of *qi* stored in the body. He himself practices Taoist breathing techniques more than any other form of exercises, and he recommends that both his students and his patients do the same. *Qi* is the body's great energiser: it controls the production of the other vital substances (blood, vital-essence, and fluid) and is involved in every vital function. Since *qi* itself is regulated with breath control, proper breathing is thus the best way to "cultivate *qi*" and constitutes the best form of preventive medicine. A man of few words, Hong Yixiang simply states, "Breathing is best."

Another aspect of kung-fu which Dr. Hong emphasises in his medical practice is physical exercise. Like Hua Tuo nearly 2,000 years before him, Hong Yixiang has developed a series

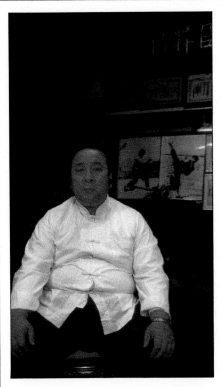

of exercises based on the fighting forms of various animals in nature. These forms adhere to the soft path of Chinese kung-fu, each move flowing smoothly from the last and melting gracefully into the next. His students must practise these forms over and over again under his watchful eye until they are "soft and natural." Based on the animal forms he teaches, he also extracts and simplifies a few basic movements which can be practised by his untrained patients. He prescribes these exercises for a wide variety of ailments: rheumatism and arthritis, nervous disorders, digestive problems, energy and blood stagnation, chronic fatigue, muscular aches, hypertension, and many more.

In addition to the animal forms, Dr. Hong is also a great proponent and master of *tai ji quan*, the classical Chinese exercise system for maintaining health and prolonging life. This is one form of Chinese therapy which has gained some acceptance in the West in recent years. *Tai ji quan* consists of a series of thirty to sixty-four smooth, rhythmic movements which must be executed with a thoroughly relaxed body, an uncluttered mind, and correct rhythmic breathing. As a means of self-defense, it is ultimately the most devastating of all forms, but it also is

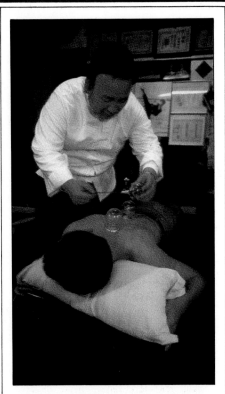

the most difficult of all to master, requiring decades of dedicated devotion. As an effective form of exercise and preventive medicine, however, *tai ji quan* can be easily learned and practised by anyone, young and old, man and woman, weak and strong alike.

Just as Dr. Huang draws from the vast store of herbal knowledge to create his own new secret prescriptions, so Dr. Hong draws from the many styles and forms established by past masters of the martial arts to create his own original style. The breathing and other therapeutic exercises which he has developed are every bit as effective as herbs, massage, acupuncture, and other more conventional forms of Chinese therapy.

Unlike Dr. Huang, Dr. Hong does not devote his entire life to serving society, for he is a Taoist and Taoists are devoted only to the Tao itself. Since his interest led him to choose the Tao of the medical and martial arts, he is totally devoted to and immersed in those arts. While Dr. Huang practises medicine for the benefit of society, Dr. Hong practises the medical and martial arts for the advancement of the arts themselves. He does not seek students for his kung-fu class or patients for his clinic, he lets them stumble upon him

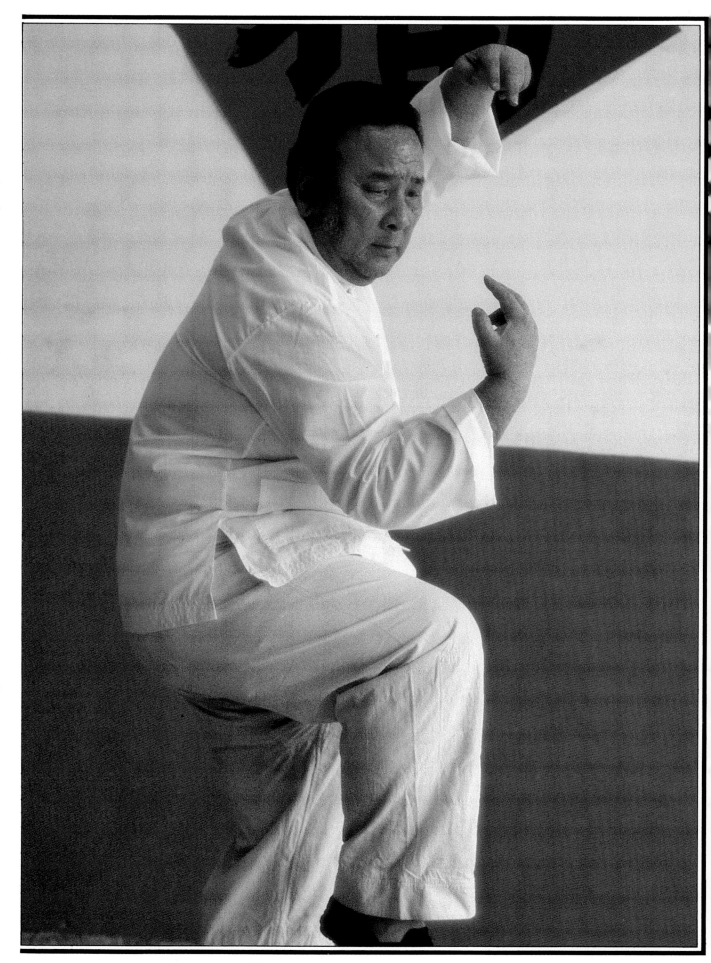

by chance. One gets the impression that he teaches students and treats patients as a side-line, preferring in fact to spend his time practising breathing and kung-fu forms, dabbling with esoteric medical techniques, and simply pondering the profundities of the Tao. Until a few years ago, he even refused to join Taiwan's Chinese Kung-fu Association, regarding all such social organisations as bothersome bores. He does not hesitate to turn away a potential student or patient whom he intuitively dislikes or feels is unworthy of his attention. He is a direct descendant of the gruff, independent mountain recluses who gave such great creative impetus to the development of Chinese medicine, a truly traditional Taoist eccentric, who is living amidst the hustle and bustle of modern Taipei, yet remains oblivious to it.

There are many such Chinese doctors practising today, especially in East Asia, where overseas Chinese communities flourish and traditional Chinese medicine is generally respected. Usually the only way to find such competent Chinese doctors is by word of mouth, for the best of them are modest, retiring people, totally devoted to the art of healing. They rarely advertise or tout their services—they don't have to. Like the Lebanese tycoon described earlier, you may well have to journey to the East to find the best Chinese healers. While there are plenty of qualified Chinese herbalists practising in the West, current laws prohibit even the most qualified Chinese doctors from practising medicine in Western countries—unless they pass Western medical examinations and qualify for Western medical licenses. Unfortunately this deprives patients in the West of the benefits of the world's oldest, safest, and in many cases, most effective medical treatments.

OPPOSITE and RIGHT *Tai ji*, the therapeutic variety of kung-fu, is practised daily by millions of people throughout China as an aid to both physical and mental health.

THE MEETING OF EAST AND WEST: THE "NEW MEDICINE"

There are several important instances of Western medicine borrowing from Chinese herbal medicine but examples are often not duly credited. Reference to New Medicine has been made earlier in this chapter. It is the only hope for up-dating the technological backwardness of traditional Chinese medicine without sacrificing its sound principles and effective practical applications. Similarly, it is the only hope for

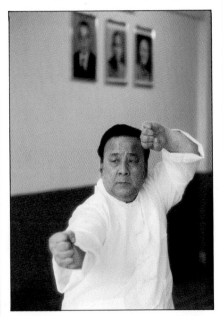

salvaging Western medical treatment from the blind excesses of "pure science" while still utilising its technological superiority. A theoretical case in point for the meeting of East and West in the field of New Medicine can be built around the recent Western discovery of the incredible disease-preventing agent interferon*.

Interferon is first and foremost a natural substance, produced in minute microscopic quantities by certain types of cells in the body. As a natural substance, a sort of "vital essence," it thus meets the first requirement of Chinese medicine: it comes directly from nature. As a microscopic molecule produced by the nuclei of living cells, however, it requires the sophistication of the most advanced Western technology to identify and isolate it. Interferon

gives credibility to the ancient Chinese premise that the key to preventing and curing disease lies inside the body and that external agents should only be used to stimulate the body's natural disease-fighting mechanisms to cure itself. Yet without modern Western technology, the specific mechanics of this premise would never have been known.

* See *Time* magazine's cover story March 31, 1980

In the case of interferon, the parallels between ancient Chinese theories and modern Western findings are remarkable. Western researchers

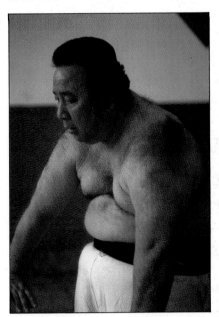

have established that interferon is produced in the body by three types of cells. The first are leukocytes or white blood cells. The second are fibroblasts, special cells which form fibrous connective tissue. And the third type are T-lymphocytes, cells which are part of the body's immunity system and produce a type of interferon which works directly with DNA master-molecules in transcribing genetic messages. A careful look at these findings will reveal profound similarities to the theories of the ancient Chinese physicians.

In our discussion of "*Qi* and the Four Vital Bodily Humours" in Chapter Three, we saw that *qi*, blood, fluid, and vital-essence are the four vital substances which Chinese medical theory cites as essential to maintaining health and prolonging life. Note, therefore, that the first

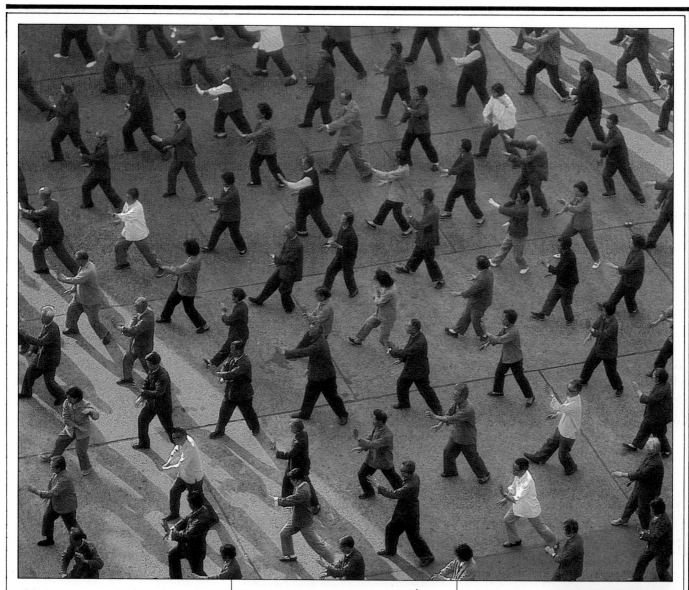

type of cell which produces interferon, white blood cells, is found in the blood, one of the vital bodily humours. The second type corresponds directly to what the Chinese describe as fluid which "lubricates the sinews and joints" and "tempers the skin and flesh," i.e. forms supple connective tissue in skin, bones, muscles, joints, and sinews.

The third type of interferon, which transcribes genetic messages and is related to the body's immunity system, is to be found in the vital

bodily-humour "vital-essence." Vital-essence includes all the vital hormones, both sexual and other, which protect the body from disease and retard the aging process. Recall as well that German scientists have proven that men with dense semen and high sperm-count, displaying strong vital-essence, are completely immune to many diseases, and highly resistant to others. This correlation between high resistance and high hormone levels has been known to the Chinese for millennia.

While the ancient Chinese had no knowledge of interferon or any other microscopic molecule, they nevertheless correctly identified those vital bodily substances capable of producing interferon. Since traditional Chinese preventive therapy prescribes constant nourishment and tonification of the vital bodily humours, it

ABOVE and RIGHT mass *tai ji* exercises on The Bund, the famous waterfront of Shanghai.

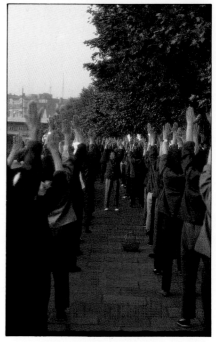

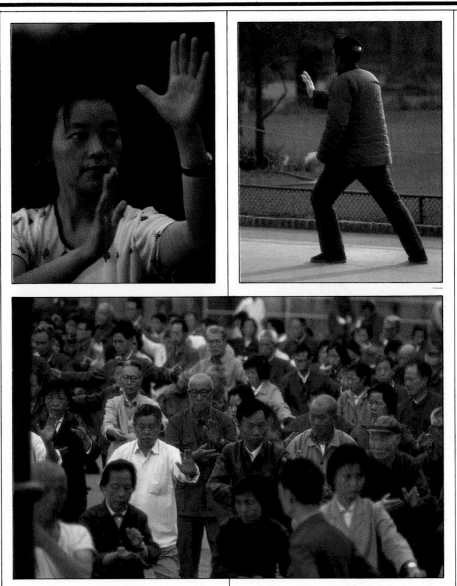

benefits of proper breathing.

The logic of the Chinese medical system indicates that interferon production in the body can be greatly enhanced by cultivating *qi*, the regulator of the three vital substances which are capable of producing interferon. *Qi* is best cultivated through correct breathing. Should proper breathing indeed prove to have this capacity, it certainly would revolutionise Western medical concepts. In light of China's past achievements in the medical field, it would seem that this aspect of Chinese therapy merits further attention in Western medical scientific circles. It is due time for Western science to take a serious look at the concept of *qi* and to bring its formidable technological resources to bear upon the problem.

The potential for further meetings of East and West in the field of medicine is exciting indeed. Currently, the initative is up to the West. The East has already embarked upon the syncretic, hybrid path of the New Medicine, which is rapidly taking root in China, Japan, and elsewhere in Asia. There is such a vast collection of Chinese medical materials to be investigated under the light of modern medical technology that researchers East and West could be kept busy for many decades to come.

In this shrinking and ever more interdependent world, there is no further excuse for the Western medical establishment to continue neglecting the profound medical discoveries of the world's oldest, most sophisticated civilisation. Such continued lack of attention to Chinese medical alternatives, whether for reasons of ignorance or professional jealousy, is tantamount to professional negligence, for Western doctors owe their patients the opportunity to benefit from Chinese treatments in those many cases where they have proved time and again to be superior to Western alternatives.

* *Science News*, 6 September, 1975

stands to reason that Chinese therapy increases the body's ability to produce interferon. Without knowing specifically why it works, the Chinese have always known exactly how to improve the body's disease-fighting and life-prolonging mechanisms.

This brings us to the problem of the most vital of all bodily humours —*qi*. According to the Chinese system, *qi* regulates the production of the other three substances and is itself the greatest of all protectors of health and life. *Qi*, however, is not recognised at all by Western medical science, and therefore no accurate correlations between East and West can be drawn on this point. But at least the West is beginning to realise that breathing involves far more than the simple exchange of oxygen and carbon dioxide in the blood. An article entitled "The Role of Lungs Expanding: Air Sacs to Endocrine Glands,"* in which some initial findings on the relationship between breath control, *qi*, and hormone production, vital-essence, are discussed. This would seem to verify the Chinese idea that *qi* regulates the production of vital-essence.

Is it possible that the Chinese have been so accurate about so many medical phenomena but wrong about the most fundamental of all their concepts? Unlikely. The evidence seems to indicate that they are right about the role of *qi* and the role of correct breathing in "cultivating *qi*". In every corner of the Orient, from Istanbul to Tokyo, doctors, yogis, martial artists, monks, philosophers, and other enlightened souls have consistently agreed upon the fundamental health-and-life-promoting

ABOVE Solitary *tai ji* exercises and "morning mass" in Shanghai park.

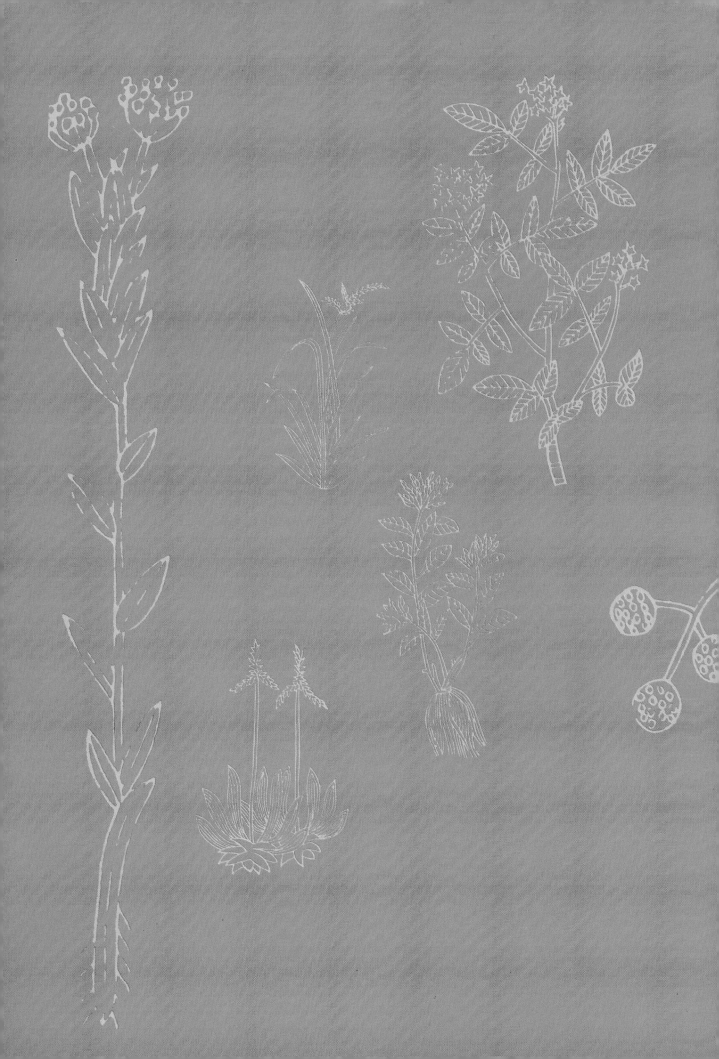

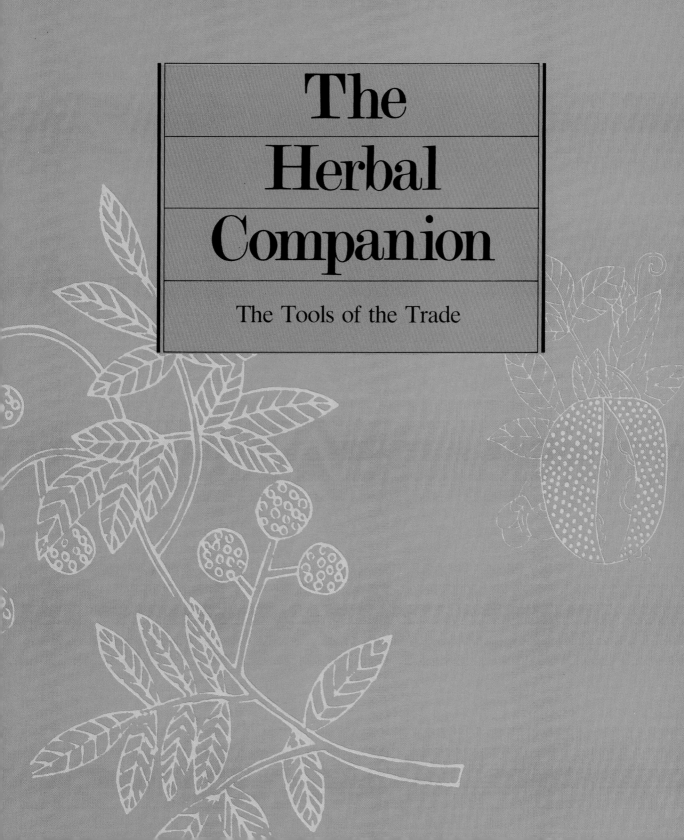

Chapter VI

The Herbal Companion

The Tools of the Trade

he Ming physician Li Shizhen listed 1892 items in his great herbal pharmacopoeia *General Outlines and Divisions of the Ben Cao (Ben Cao Gang Mu)*. The bulk of these items, however, are seldom used in normal practice or are employed only when other more common ingredients are unavailable. Many are rare, exotic tonics, which are not needed in ordinary preventive and curative prescription and which only the very

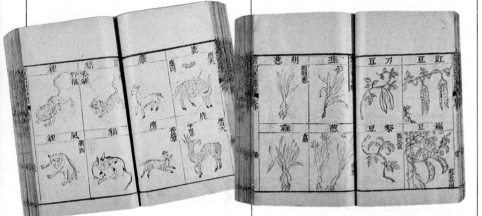

wealthy can afford. About 300 varieties of herbal ingredients are commonly used in preparing prescriptions, and of those, about 150 are considered vital, indispensable components. In order to provide more detailed descriptions of each item, we restrict our discussion here to these but, to round off our presentation, include some of the more unusual, esoteric items. Most of the essential and frequently used ingredients can be readily obtained in Chinese herb shops around the world.

Following the example of many Chinese herbal handbooks, the herbs described below are arranged in groups according to their essential functional effects, rather than botanical or zoological types. This is the practical approach used by most practising Chinese herbalists: all drugs which take essentially similar action and direction in the body are listed under the same headings, such as "purgatives," "demulcents," "tonics," etc. Under this arrangement, plant, animal, and mineral derivatives with similar effects appear together under the appropriate headings. Each functional group of herbs listed is preceded by a brief description of the

group's general effects and uses.

Each herbal item is described according to the following outline:
— Latin botanical name and family name
— Common English name, if available
— Chinese name, romanised and in Chinese characters
— Natural distribution
— Parts used
— Nature: essential flavour; essential energy
— Natural affinity: organs and meridians affected
— Essential pharmacodynamic effects
— Chinese therapeutic uses
— Average daily dosage (when used singly as decoction or infusion)
— Remarks

After the herbal descriptions, a list of common herbal prescriptions in which they appear is presented. These prescriptions have been gleaned from ancient Chinese herbal manuals as well as contemporary Chinese herbal practice. They are not meant to be viewed as magic panaceas for every ill, but rather as examples of how the tools of the herbalist's trade are employed in practical applications. When properly prepared with good ingredients and used for the purposes described, these prescriptions are perfectly safe and effective remedies. It is always best, however, to consult a Chinese doctor or herbalist before embarking on herbal treatments.

The following Western medical terms appear in the descriptions of the herb's pharmacodynamic effects:

Analgesic: producing a state of not feeling pain while retaining full consciousness and other sensations

Anaesthetic: producing a state of not feeling pain or any other sensation; in general anaesthesia, loss of consciousness is induced
Anthelmintic: killing and/or ejecting intestinal worms and parasites
Antidote: counteracting poisons and other toxic substances
Antiphlogistic: counteracting inflammation
Antipyretic: reducing fever
Antiseptic: killing or inhibiting the action of microorganisms (germs)
Antispasmodic: relieving or preventing spasms
Antitussive: reducing the severity and frequency of coughs
Aphrodisiac: arousing or increasing sexual desire
Astringent, styptic: contracting body tissue and blood vessels to check the flow of blood
Carminative: causing gas to be expelled from the stomach and intestines
Cathartic: inducing the evacuation of the bowels; medium-strength
Demulcent: soothing irritated or inflamed mucous membranes
Diaphoretic: inducing or increasing perspiration
Digestive: aiding digestion and distribution of nutrients
Diuretic: increasing the secretion and flow of urine
Emmenagogue: stimulating the menstrual flow
Emollient: softening; soothing
Expectorant: causing or easing the bringing up of phlegm, mucus, and sputum from the respiratory tract
Emetic: inducing vomiting
Hemostatic: stopping the flow of blood
Laxative: inducing the evacuation of the bowels; mild form
Purgative: inducing the evacuation of the bowels; strong, drastic form
Refrigerant: cooling and reducing heat and fever
Sedative: tending to soothe and reduce excitement, nervousness, irritation, and other forms of over-stimulation
Stimulant: increasing the activity of vital processes and organs
Stomachic: tonifying the stomach to improve digestive functions
Tonic: restoring or increasing muscular tone of damaged or weak tissues; stimulating vitality; promoting vital functions

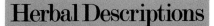

Herbal Descriptions

DIAPHORETIC OR "RELEASE EXTERNALLY"

Diaphoretic medicines are those which induce or increase perspiration in order to release "evil-*qi*" in cases of external ailments, such as exposure to excess wind, rain, or heat. *The Internal Book of Huang Di* states, "If it's in the skin, sweat it out." These herbs are most effective in the initial stages of such ailments, before they have moved inward.

Diaphoretics are generally pungent and warm by nature and tend to scatter *qi*. Used in excess, they have adverse effects on fluid balance and yang-energy. There are two types: those used to dispel "wind-cold" and those used to dispel "wind-heat" symptoms.

1

EPHEDRA SINICA
(Gnetaceae)

JOINT FIR

麻黄

ma huang

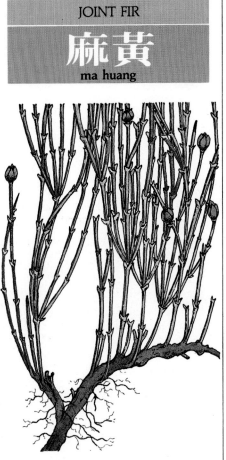

Natural distribution: Northern China, Mongolia, Europe
Parts used: Stems
Nature: Pungent and slightly bitter; warm
Affinity: Lungs, bladder
Effects: Diaphoretic; stimulant to respiration; dilate bronchi; diuretic
Indications: "Wind-cold" chills and fever; bronchial asthma; hay fever
Dosage: 3-10 g
Remarks: For asthma use with almond; for "wind-cold" injury use with cinnamon; for allergic skin reaction use with mint and cicada moltings. Roots are anti-diaphoretic

---

2

CINNAMOMUM CASSIA
(Lauraceae)

CINNAMON TREE

桂枝

gui zhi

Natural distribution: Southern China, Laos, Vietnam
Parts used: Tender young stems
Nature: Pungent and sweet; warm
Affinity: Heart, lungs, bladder
Effects: Diaphoretic; carminative; antiseptic; emmenagogue
Indications: "Wind-cold" chills and fever; diarrhoea; nausea; menstrual disorders
Dosage: 1-5 g
Remarks: Fevers without sweat, use with *Ephedra sinica*; with sweat, use with *Paeonia albiflora*; for menstrual disorders, use with *Paeonia lactiflora*, *Prunus persica*, and *Angelica sinensis*

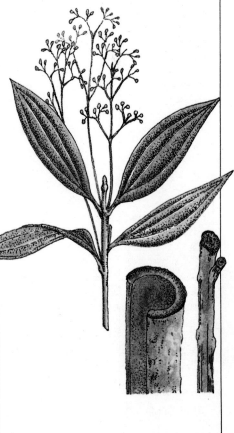

81

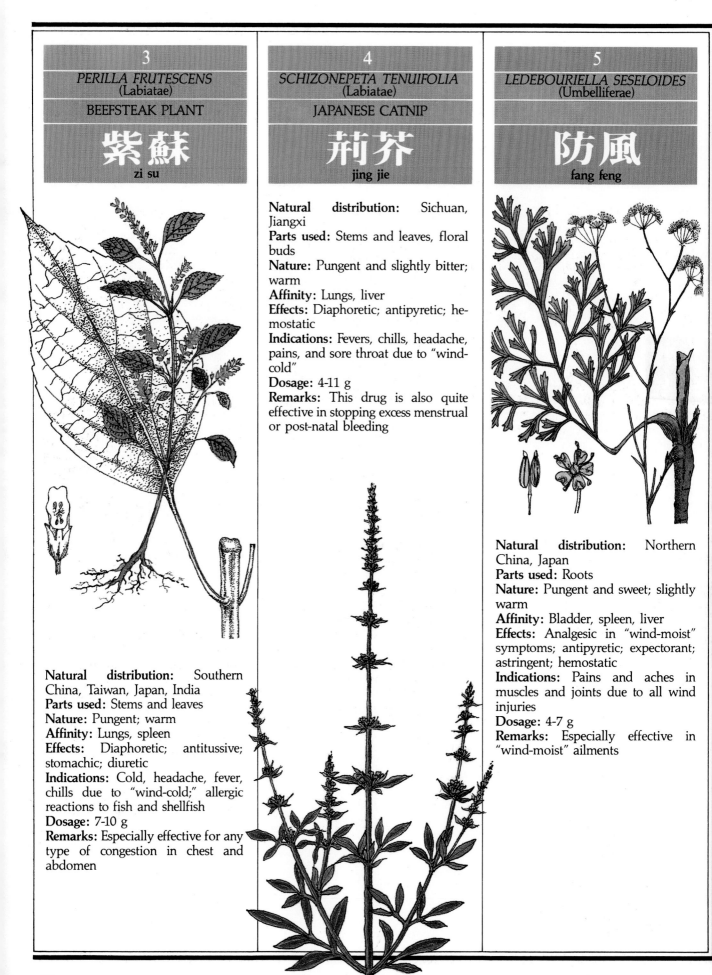

3	4	5
PERILLA FRUTESCENS (Labiatae) BEEFSTEAK PLANT	*SCHIZONEPETA TENUIFOLIA* (Labiatae) JAPANESE CATNIP	*LEDEBOURIELLA SESELOIDES* (Umbelliferae)

3 — 紫蘇 zi su

Natural distribution: Southern China, Taiwan, Japan, India
Parts used: Stems and leaves
Nature: Pungent; warm
Affinity: Lungs, spleen
Effects: Diaphoretic; antitussive; stomachic; diuretic
Indications: Cold, headache, fever, chills due to "wind-cold;" allergic reactions to fish and shellfish
Dosage: 7-10 g
Remarks: Especially effective for any type of congestion in chest and abdomen

4 — 荆芥 jing jie

Natural distribution: Sichuan, Jiangxi
Parts used: Stems and leaves, floral buds
Nature: Pungent and slightly bitter; warm
Affinity: Lungs, liver
Effects: Diaphoretic; antipyretic; hemostatic
Indications: Fevers, chills, headache, pains, and sore throat due to "wind-cold"
Dosage: 4-11 g
Remarks: This drug is also quite effective in stopping excess menstrual or post-natal bleeding

5 — 防風 fang feng

Natural distribution: Northern China, Japan
Parts used: Roots
Nature: Pungent and sweet; slightly warm
Affinity: Bladder, spleen, liver
Effects: Analgesic in "wind-moist" symptoms; antipyretic; expectorant; astringent; hemostatic
Indications: Pains and aches in muscles and joints due to all wind injuries
Dosage: 4-7 g
Remarks: Especially effective in "wind-moist" ailments

6

ASARUM SIEBOLDII
(Aristolochiaceae)

細辛
xi xin

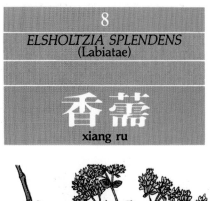

Natural distribution: Northern China, Japan

Parts used: Whole plant, roots are best

Nature: Pungent; warm

Affinity: Heart, lungs, liver, kidneys

Effects: Diaphoretic; expectorant; sedative; analgesic

Indications: All types of colds, fevers, chills, and headaches

Dosage: 2-5 g

Remarks: Effective relief for all types of pain in the head, including acute toothaches; the powdered herb is stuffed into the navel to eliminate abscesses in the mouth

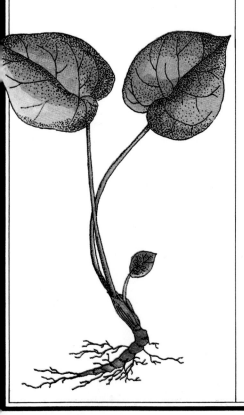

7

ANGELICA ANOMALA
(Umbelliferae)

白芷
bai zhi

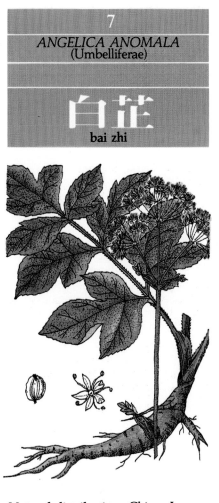

Natural distribution: China, Japan

Parts used: Roots

Nature: Pungent and bitter; warm

Affinity: Lungs, stomach

Effects: Analgesic in wind-injury; reduces swelling; antidote

Indications: Colds, headaches, aches and pains due to wind-injury; abscesses and swelling; leucorrhoea; congestion; snake-bites

Dosage: 4-7 g

Remarks: Important ingredient in antidote potions for poisonous snake-bites

8

ELSHOLTZIA SPLENDENS
(Labiatae)

香薷
xiang ru

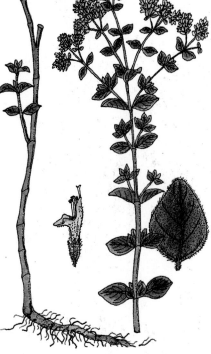

Natural distribution: China, Japan, Korea, Vietnam, Laos

Parts used: Whole plant, with flowers

Nature: Pungent; slightly warm

Affinity: Lungs, stomach

Effects: Diaphoretic; carminative; stomachic; diuretic

Indications: Ailments and swelling from "moist-excess;" "wind-cold" injuries; summer chills; nausea and diarrhoea

Dosage: 4-8 g

Remarks: This herb is also used to eliminate bad breath

9

ALLIUM FISTULOSUM
(Liliaceae)

CHINESE "SPRING ONIONS"

葱白
cong bai

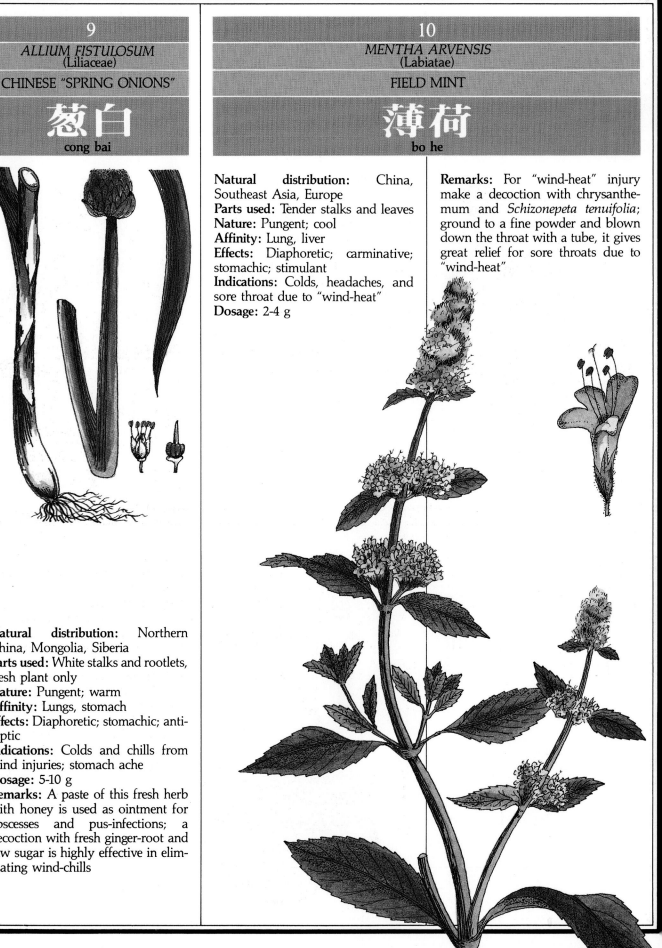

Natural distribution: Northern China, Mongolia, Siberia
Parts used: White stalks and rootlets, fresh plant only
Nature: Pungent; warm
Affinity: Lungs, stomach
Effects: Diaphoretic; stomachic; antiseptic
Indications: Colds and chills from wind injuries; stomach ache
Dosage: 5-10 g
Remarks: A paste of this fresh herb with honey is used as ointment for abscesses and pus-infections; a decoction with fresh ginger-root and raw sugar is highly effective in eliminating wind-chills

10

MENTHA ARVENSIS
(Labiatae)

FIELD MINT

薄荷
bo he

Natural distribution: China, Southeast Asia, Europe
Parts used: Tender stalks and leaves
Nature: Pungent; cool
Affinity: Lung, liver
Effects: Diaphoretic; carminative; stomachic; stimulant
Indications: Colds, headaches, and sore throat due to "wind-heat"
Dosage: 2-4 g

Remarks: For "wind-heat" injury make a decoction with chrysanthemum and *Schizonepeta tenuifolia*; ground to a fine powder and blown down the throat with a tube, it gives great relief for sore throats due to "wind-heat"

11

MAGNOLIA LILIFLORA
(Magnoliaceae)

MAGNOLIA TREE

辛夷

xin yi

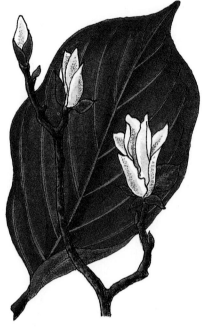

Natural distribution: China, Japan
Parts used: Unopened floral buds
Nature: Pungent; warm
Affinity: Lungs, stomach
Effects: Analgesic; decongestant
Indications: All ailments of the nose; sinusitis
Dosage: 5-8 g
Remarks: Incompatible with *Astragalus membranaceus*

12

ARCTIUM LAPPA
(Compositae)

GREAT BURDOCK

牛蒡子

niu bang zi

Natural distribution: Northern China, Europe
Parts used: Seeds, sometimes the root
Nature: Pungent and bitter; cold
Affinity: Lungs, stomach
Effects: Antipyretic; antiphlogistic; diuretic; expectorant; anti-toxic
Indications: All "wind-heat" ailments; throat infections; pneumonia; inflammations of urinal tract; abscesses
Dosage: 3-10 g
Remarks: A tincture of the seed applied topically is effective in curing psoriasis inveterata, hemorrhoids, and chronic sores

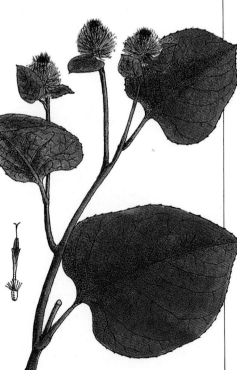

13

MORUS ALBA
(Moraceae)

WHITE MULBERRY TREE

桑葉

sang ye

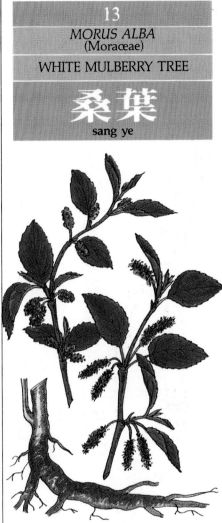

Natural distribution: China, Japan, Southeast Asia
Parts used: Leaves
Nature: Bitter and sweet; cold
Affinity: Lungs, liver
Effects: Antipyretic; sedative to liver; improves vision; refrigerant
Indications: Colds, headache and coughs due to "wind-heat" injury; swelling and pain in the eyes
Dosage: 5-10 g
Remarks: The root is used as an antitussive and expectorant in asthma, bronchitis, and coughs

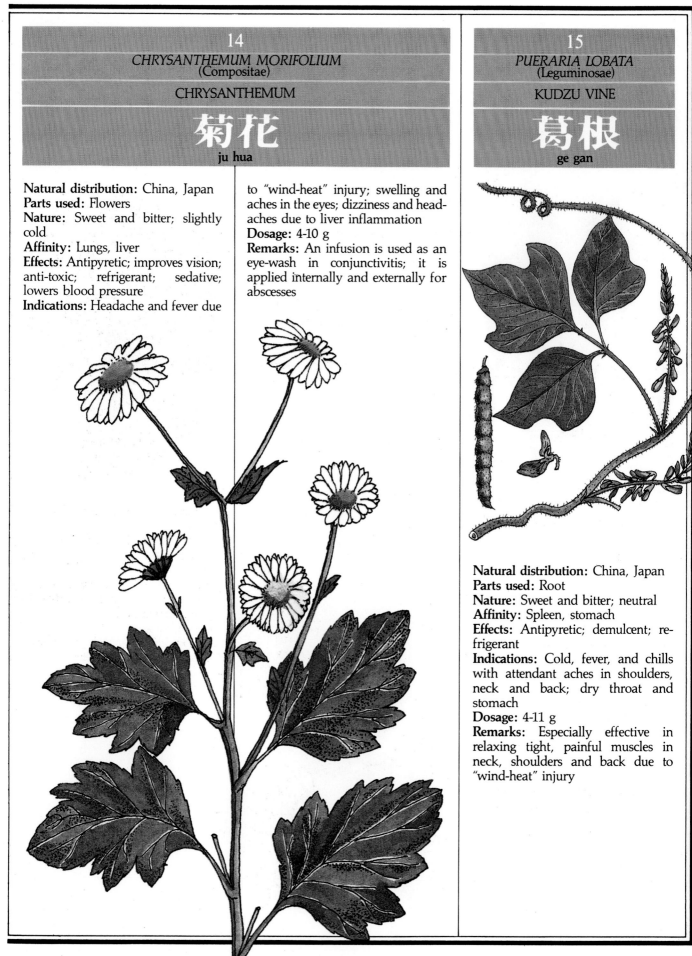

14
CHRYSANTHEMUM MORIFOLIUM
(Compositae)

CHRYSANTHEMUM

菊花
ju hua

Natural distribution: China, Japan
Parts used: Flowers
Nature: Sweet and bitter; slightly cold
Affinity: Lungs, liver
Effects: Antipyretic; improves vision; anti-toxic; refrigerant; sedative; lowers blood pressure
Indications: Headache and fever due to "wind-heat" injury; swelling and aches in the eyes; dizziness and headaches due to liver inflammation
Dosage: 4-10 g
Remarks: An infusion is used as an eye-wash in conjunctivitis; it is applied internally and externally for abscesses

15
PUERARIA LOBATA
(Leguminosae)

KUDZU VINE

葛根
ge gan

Natural distribution: China, Japan
Parts used: Root
Nature: Sweet and bitter; neutral
Affinity: Spleen, stomach
Effects: Antipyretic; demulcent; refrigerant
Indications: Cold, fever, and chills with attendant aches in shoulders, neck and back; dry throat and stomach
Dosage: 4-11 g
Remarks: Especially effective in relaxing tight, painful muscles in neck, shoulders and back due to "wind-heat" injury

16	17	18

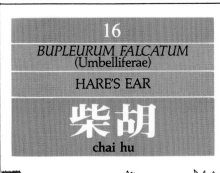

BUPLEURUM FALCATUM
(Umbelliferae)

HARE'S EAR

柴胡
chai hu

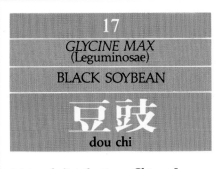

GLYCINE MAX
(Leguminosae)

BLACK SOYBEAN

豆豉
dou chi

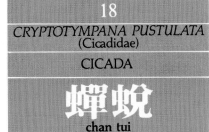

CRYPTOTYMPANA PUSTULATA
(Cicadidae)

CICADA

蟬蛻
chan tui

Natural distribution: China, Japan
Parts used: Seeds (beans) of black variety
Nature: Sweet and slightly bitter; cold
Affinity: Lung, stomach
Effects: Carminative; sedative; antipyretic
Indications: Colds, fevers, and headaches due to "wind-heat" injury; oppression in chest; insomnia
Dosage: 10-15 g
Remarks: Black soybeans must be fermented before becoming medically useful

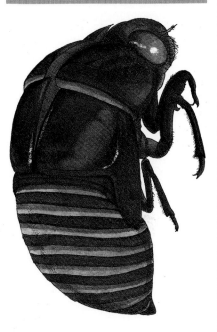

Natural distribution: China, Taiwan, Japan
Parts used: Exuviae (molting)
Nature: Sweet; cold
Affinity: Lungs, liver
Effects: Antipyretic; antispasmodic
Indications: Cataracts; "wind-heat" injuries; convulsions
Dosage: 3-5 g
Remarks: For cataracts, mix with *Chrysanthemum morifolium*

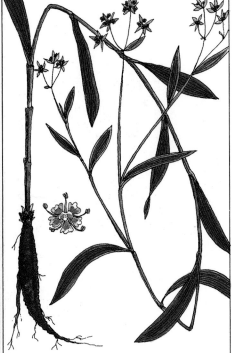

Natural distribution: Northern China, northern Europe
Parts used: Root
Nature: Bitter; neutral
Affinity: Pericardium, liver, triplewarmer, gall bladder
Effects: Antipyretic; sedative to liver
Indications: Intermittant fevers and chills; malaria; blackwater fever
Dosage: 2-5 g
Remarks: This herb is quite effective in treating prolapse of internal organs such as rectum, womb, etc.

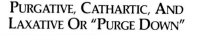

PURGATIVE, CATHARTIC, AND LAXATIVE OR "PURGE DOWN"

All herbs which induce evacuation of the bowels fall into this category. The strong, fast-acting drugs which purge drastically are called purgative; medium-strength herbs are called cathartic; and mild, gentle drugs which act mainly by lubrication of the large intestine are referred to as laxative. In addition to various other organs, these herbs all have a strong affinity for the large intestine and/or its connected organ, the lungs.

These medications have three basic effects: they induce or facilitate loose bowel movements in order to eliminate stagnant food and accumulated faeces from the intestinal tract; they tend to "clear heat" and "purge fire" from the system by forcing these excesses out through the bowels with the faeces; they expel excess liquids and reduce swelling by driving out "water-evil" through the faeces and urine.

Strong purgatives should only be used for acute constipation in strong, otherwise healthy patients. Cathartics and laxatives are more appropriate for chronic constipation, as well as children, the elderly, and the weak.

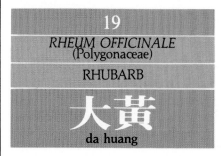

19
RHEUM OFFICINALE
(Polygonaceae)

RHUBARB

大黃
da huang

Natural distribution: Western China, Tibet
Parts used: Rhizomes
Nature: Bitter; cold
Affinity: Spleen, stomach, large intestine, pericardium, liver
Effects: Purgative (2-5 g); laxative (1-2 g); astringent (0.3 g) refrigerant; emmenagogue
Indications: Constipation; amenorrhoea; eye pressure from liver inflammation; energy and blood stagnation due to traumatic injury
Dosage: see above
Remarks: The powdered herb applied to burns relieves pain and swelling

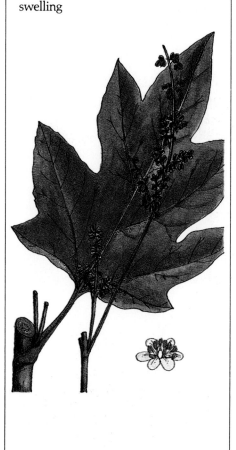

20
MIRABILITE
(Sodium Sulfate Decahydrate)

GLAUBER'S SALT

芒硝
mang xiao

Natural distribution: Common world-wide
Parts used: Crystals
Nature: Salty, pungent and bitter; very cold
Affinity: Stomach, large intestine, triple-warmer
Effects: Purgative
Indications: Constipation due to heat excess
Dosage: 10-18 g
Remarks: Used with *Rheum officinale* for constipation; used as eye wash and gargle for heat excess symptoms and on abscesses; the powdered drug is rubbed on the nipples to wean children from breast-feeding; a paste of this drug with *Rheum officinale* and fresh garlic cloves is taped tightly over the appendix in cases of acute appendicitis

21	22	23
CASSIA ANGUSTIFOLIA (Leguminosae)	*ALOE BARBADENSIS* (Liliaceae)	*CANNABIS SATIVA* (Cannabinaceae)
TINNEVELLY SENNA	BARBADOS or CURACAO ALOE	HEMP
番瀉葉 fan xie ye	蘆薈 lu hui	火麻仁 huo ma ren

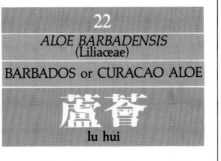

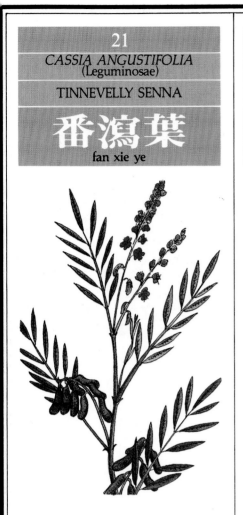

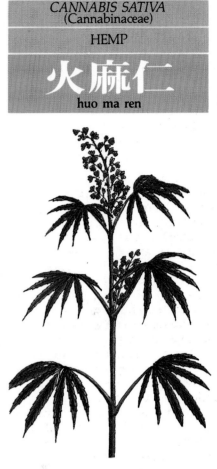

Natural distribution: Western Africa, West Indies, India
Parts used: Condensed juice of the fresh leaves
Nature: Bitter; cold
Affinity: Liver, stomach, large intestine
Effects: Purgative (0.3-1 g); laxative (0.06-0.2 g);
Indications: stomachic (0.01-0.03 g); refrigerant; antiseptic; emmenagogue; sedative to liver Chronic constipation; dizziness, headache and delirium due to liver inflammations; intestinal parasites
Dosage: 0.01-1 g
Remarks: Does not lose effect with prolonged use, so is good for chronic cases of constipation

Natural distribution: India, Arabia, Africa
Parts used: Leaflets
Nature: Sweet and bitter; very cold
Affinity: Large intestine
Effects: Purgative (4-8 g); cathartic (1-3 g); laxative (0.5-1 g)
Indications: Constipation from heat excess
Dosage: see above
Remarks: Doses over 5 g may cause unpleasant symptoms of nausea, vomiting and stomach ache

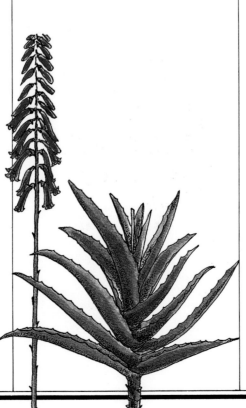

Natural distribution: China, India, Afghanistan, Indochina, North Africa
Parts used: Seeds
Nature: Sweet; neutral
Affinity: Spleen, stomach, large intestine
Effects: Laxative; emollient; demulcent; antitussive; antiseptic; antidote
Indications: Constipation due to fluid deficiency, especially in old age and post-natal
Dosage: 11 g
Remarks: Every part is used in medicine; the stalk is diuretic; the oil is demulcent for dry throat; the male flowers are used in wind-injury and menstrual disorders; the resinous female flowers are slightly poisonous, are stimulant to the central nervous system, and are used in nervous disorders; used in excess, remarks Li Shizhen, the latter will induce "hallucinations and an unsteady gait."

24	25	26

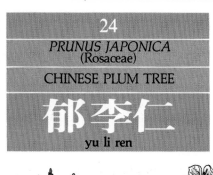

24
PRUNUS JAPONICA
(Rosaceae)
CHINESE PLUM TREE
郁李仁
yu li ren

25
APIS MELLIFERA
(Apidae)
HONEY
蜂蜜
feng mi

26
EUPHORBIA KANSUI
(Euphorbiaceae)
甘遂
gan sui

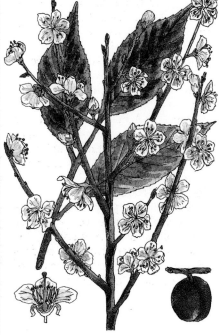

Natural distribution: Common world-wide
Nature: Sweet; neutral
Affinity: Lungs, spleen, large intestine
Effects: Laxative; demulcent; nutrient; emollient in chronic bronchitis, dry throat and mouth
Dosage: 10-75 g
Indications: Remarks: Honey is the base for making most herbal pill prescriptions; should be avoided by those with chronic loose bowels

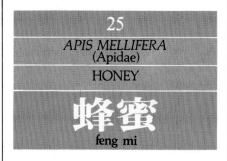

Natural distribution: Sichuan, Jiangsu
Parts used: Kernel of the seeds
Nature: Pungent, bitter and sweet; neutral
Affinity: Large intestine, small intestine, spleen
Effects: Laxative; emollient; diuretic; reduces swelling
Indications: Constipation due to fluid deficiency; water-retention
Dosage: 4-7 g
Remarks: May cause slight abdominal discomfort when taking effect against constipation

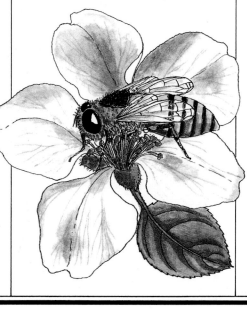

Natural distribution: China, Korea, Japan
Parts used: Roots
Nature: Bitter; cold
Affinity: Lungs, spleen, kidneys
Effects: Purgative; diuretic; reduces swelling; expectorant
Indications: Constipation; water retention; swelling; oppression in chest; epilepsy; external application for pain and numbness in muscles
Dosage: 2-4 g
Remarks: Mildy poisonous; the drug is strong and should be used cautiously; should be avoided by pregnant women, the weak and elderly

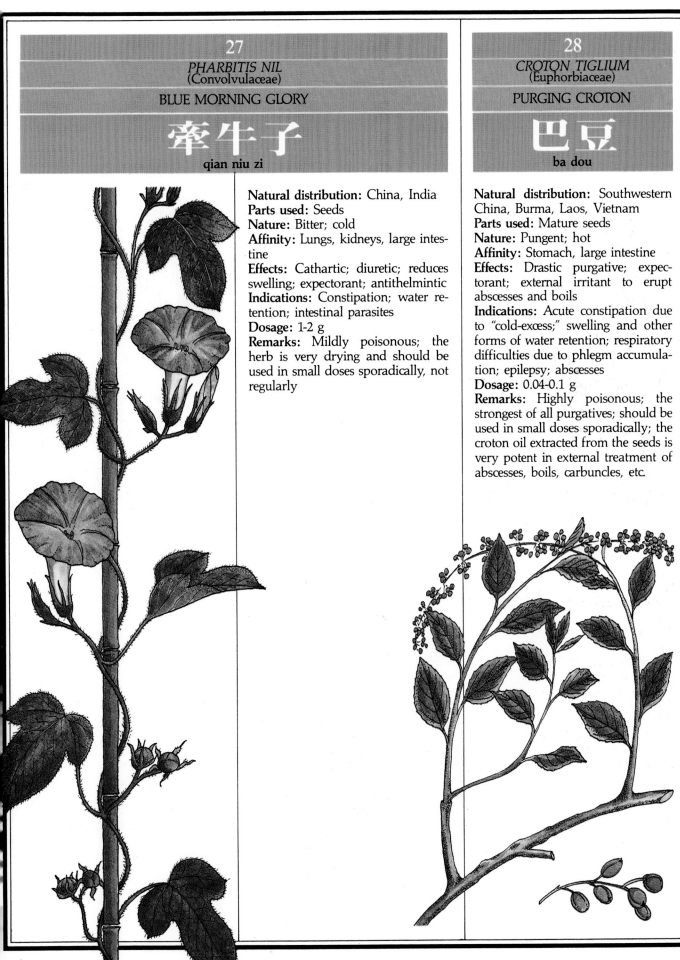

27

PHARBITIS NIL
(Convolvulaceae)

BLUE MORNING GLORY

牽牛子

qian niu zi

Natural distribution: China, India
Parts used: Seeds
Nature: Bitter; cold
Affinity: Lungs, kidneys, large intestine
Effects: Cathartic; diuretic; reduces swelling; expectorant; antithelmintic
Indications: Constipation; water retention; intestinal parasites
Dosage: 1-2 g
Remarks: Mildly poisonous; the herb is very drying and should be used in small doses sporadically, not regularly

28

CROTON TIGLIUM
(Euphorbiaceae)

PURGING CROTON

巴豆

ba dou

Natural distribution: Southwestern China, Burma, Laos, Vietnam
Parts used: Mature seeds
Nature: Pungent; hot
Affinity: Stomach, large intestine
Effects: Drastic purgative; expectorant; external irritant to erupt abscesses and boils
Indications: Acute constipation due to "cold-excess;" swelling and other forms of water retention; respiratory difficulties due to phlegm accumulation; epilepsy; abscesses
Dosage: 0.04-0.1 g
Remarks: Highly poisonous; the strongest of all purgatives; should be used in small doses sporadically; the croton oil extracted from the seeds is very potent in external treatment of abscesses, boils, carbuncles, etc.

29

GYPSUM FIBROSUM
(Calcium sulfate)

GYPSUM

石膏

shi gao

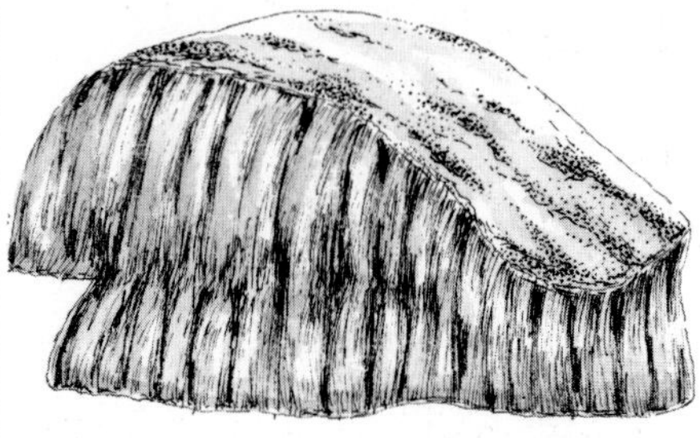

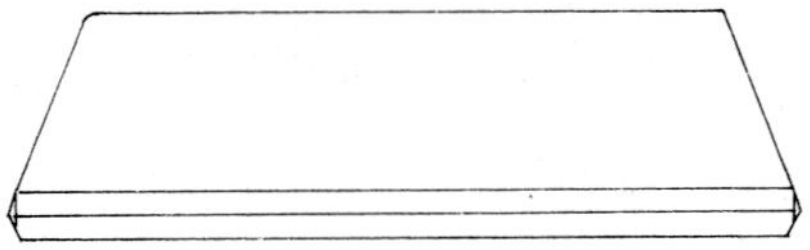

ANTIPYRETIC, REFRIGERANT OR "CLEARING HEAT"

Antipyretics and refrigerants are those drugs which "clear up internal heat." They are used against all ailments and symptoms caused by excess internal heat: dysentery, ulcers, abscesses, carbuncles, sore and swollen eyes, hot throat and parched mouth, heat-rash, liver and gland inflammations, dizziness, delirium, jaundice, insomnia, and others *The Internal Book of Huang Di* instructs, "If it's hot, cool it down."

Chinese herbal manuals distinguish six sub-categories of heat-clearing herbs:

"Purge-fire" types are used when the body is literally "over-heated" from excess "hot" and "full" conditions.

"Clear liver, brighten eyes" herbs are used against liver inflammations and attendant symptoms, such as sore, swollen, and red eyes, blurry vision, headaches, etc.

"Clear heat, cool blood" medicines go directly to the blood to "cool" down side-effects of heat excess in that vital bodily humour.

"Clear heat, expel poison" type herbs eliminate natural toxins, such as pus, produced in the body due to heat excess; they are also general antidotes.

"Clear heat, dry dampness" drugs are used against symptoms of "damp-full" and "damp-hot" excess, such as summer colds, aching joints and muscles, leukorrhoea, jaundice, etc.

"Clear empty-heat" items are used in cases of "dry-hot" excess and in heat injuries caused by blood or energy deficiency.

These drugs are all "cold" or "cool" yin medicines. Those with yang-energy deficiency and/or weak stomach and spleen should use these items sparingly.

Natural distribution: Common world-wide
Parts used: Crystal
Nature: Pungent, sweet; very cold
Affinity: Lungs, stomach
Effects: Antipyretic; antiphlogistic; astringent
Indications: Physical and emotional symptoms of heat excess: body heat, thirst, heat rash, headache, toothache; heat excess in stomach and lungs; coughs due to asthma and bronchitis; external application to abscesses and burns
Dosage: 10-35 g

30	31	32
ANEMARRHENA ASPHODELOIDES (Liliaceae)	*GARDENIA JASMINOIDES* (Rubiaceae)	*PHRAGMITES COMMUNIS* (Gramineae)
	GARDENIA	REED GRASS
知母	梔子	蘆根
zhi mu	zhi zi	lu gen

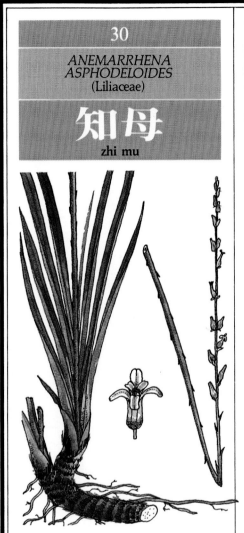

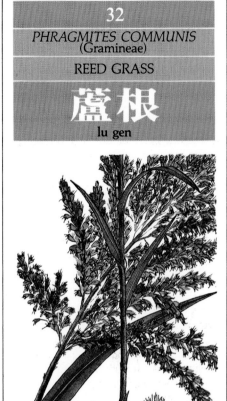

Natural distribution: China, Taiwan, Japan
Parts used: Mature fruit
Nature: Bitter; cold
Affinity: Heart, liver, lungs, stomach
Effects: Antipyretic; refrigerant to blood; antidote; antiphlogistic; hemostatic
Indications: Heat excess ailments: fever, restlessness, irritability, nosebleeds, blood in urine and sputum, swollen and sore eyes, abscesses
Dosage: 5-10 g
Remarks: A paste of the herb with flour and wine is used as poultice on twists, sprains, strains, bruises, and abscesses; very effective in injuries to tendons, ligaments, joints, and muscles

Natural distribution: Northern China
Parts used: Rhizomes and stems
Nature: Bitter; cold
Affinity: Lungs, stomach, kidneys
Effects: Antipyretic; demulcent; tonic to kidneys
Indications: Body heat, irritability, thirst, insomnia, etc. due to heat excess; pneumonia and chronic bronchitis; "yin-empty" ailments
Dosage: 3-7 g
Remarks: This drug is incompatible with iron preparations

Natural distribution: Common world-wide
Parts used: Roots and stems
Nature: Sweet; cold
Affinity: Lungs, stomach
Effects: Antipyretic; demulcent; refrigerant to stomach and lungs
Indications: Body heat, thirst and parched throat due to heat excess; vomiting due to excess stomach heat; coughing and thick, dark phlegm due to excess lung heat
Dosage: 20-40 g
Remarks: The herb is an antidote in food poisoning, especially from seafood

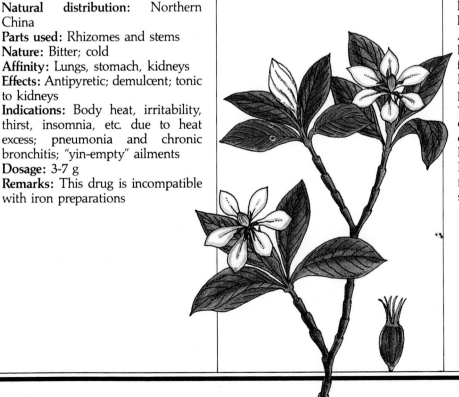

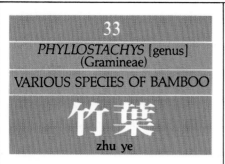

33
PHYLLOSTACHYS [genus]
(Gramineae)
VARIOUS SPECIES OF BAMBOO
竹葉
zhu ye

Natural distribution: Central China, Japan
Parts used: Leaves
Nature: Sweet; cold
Affinity: Heart, small intestine
Effects: Antipyretic; diuretic; antispasmodic
Indications: Body heat, thirst, irritability, abscesses in mouth, dark and scanty urine due to heat excess
Dosage: 10-15 g
Remarks: The fresh leaves are more effective for heat excess symptoms in stomach, heart, and parts above; the dried leaves are better for diuretic purposes

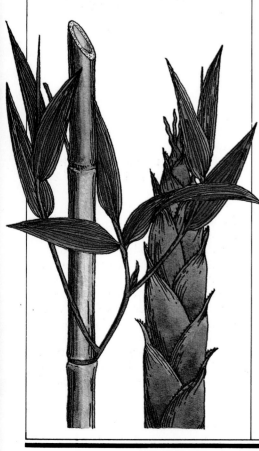

34
PRUNELLA VULGARIS
(Labiatae)
SELF-HEAL or HEAL-ALL
夏枯草
xia ku cao

Natural distribution: Northern China, northern Europe, North America
Parts used: Flowers and kernels (inflorescence)
Nature: Pungent and bitter; cold
Affinity: Liver, gall bladder
Effects: Antipyretic; refrigerant to liver; diuretic; reduces swelling of lymph glands
Indications: Jaundice; sore and swollen eyeballs; over-sensitivity to light; headache and dizziness; gout; scrofula; high blood pressure
Dosage: 5-7 g
Remarks: This drug is highly effective in all symptoms of jaundice

35
CELOSIA ARGENTEA
(Amarantaceae)
QUAIL GRASS
青葙子
qing xiang zi

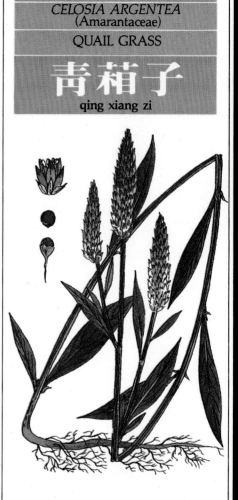

Natural distribution: Southern China, India, Sri Lanka, Africa, America
Parts used: Seeds
Nature: Bitter; slightly cold
Affinity: Liver
Effects: Antipyretic and antiphlogistic to liver; astringent in conjunctivitis
Indications: High blood pressure, all attendant eye problems
Dosage: 6-15 g
Remarks: A recent, effective new application of this drug is to mix it with Chrysanthemum and *Prunella vulgaris* for high blood pressure

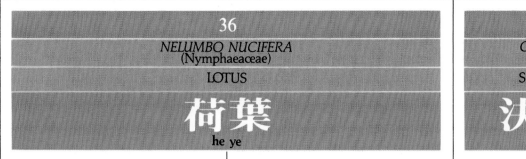

36

NELUMBO NUCIFERA
(Nymphaeaceae)

LOTUS

荷葉

he ye

Natural distribution: Asia, Australia
Parts used: Leaves
Nature: Bitter; neutral
Affinity: Liver, spleen, stomach
Effects: Antipyretic; refrigerant
Indications: Summer-heat ailments; oppression in chest; pressure in head; thirst; dark and scanty urine
Dosage: ¼ of a leaf per dose
Remarks: Every part of the lotus plant is used in medicine: the stem relieves congestion in chest due to "damp-heat" excess; the peduncle is used for stomach aches, to calm the foetus, and leukorrhoea; the seeds are used for insomnia, spermatorrhoea, and diarrhoea; the stamens are a preventive for premature ejaculation

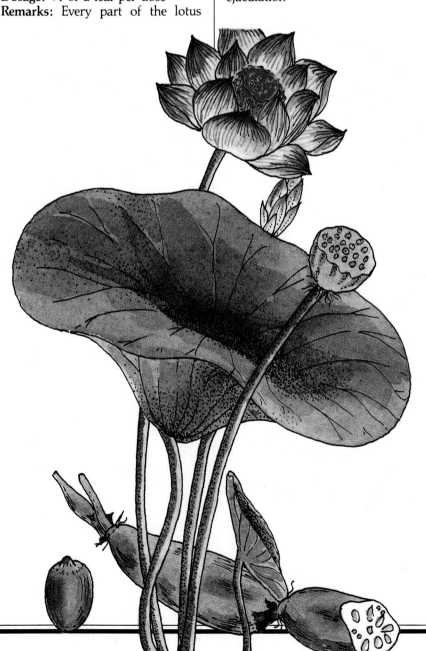

37

CASSIA TORA
(Leguminosae)

SICKLE SENNA

決明子

jue ming zi

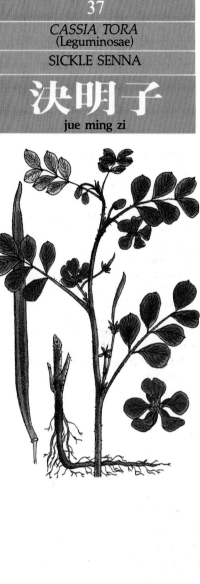

Natural distribution: Southern China, Indochina, India, Southeast Asia
Parts used: Seeds
Nature: Sweet, bitter and salty; slightly cold
Affinity: Liver, gall bladder
Effects: Antipyretic to liver; laxative; promotes clear vision
Indications: All eye problems due to liver inflammation: swelling, soreness, over-sensitivity to light, etc.
Dosage: 5-8 g
Remarks: A very natural-acting laxative; safe and effective for chronic constipation; it also lowers blood pressure effectively

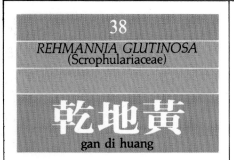

38	39	40

38

REHMANNIA GLUTINOSA
(Scrophulariaceae)

乾地黃

gan di huang

Natural distribution: Northern China

Parts used: Root

Nature: Sweet; cold

Affinity: Heart, liver, kidneys, small intestine

Effects: Antipyretic; "cools" and tonifies the blood; cardiotonic; demulcent; hemostatic; diuretic

Indications: Body heat and heat rash due to internal heat excess; yin-deficiency due to heat injuries; diabetes

Dosage: 5-8 g

Remarks: A strong cardiovascular tonic, excellent for patients with weak hearts; this drug effectively lowers blood sugar

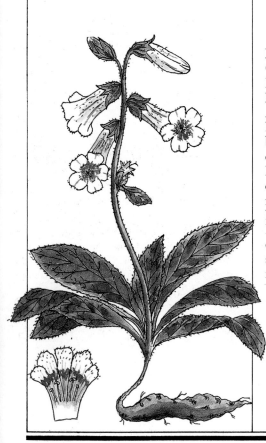

39

LITHOSPERMUM ERYTHRORHIZON
(Boraginaceae)

紫草

zi cao

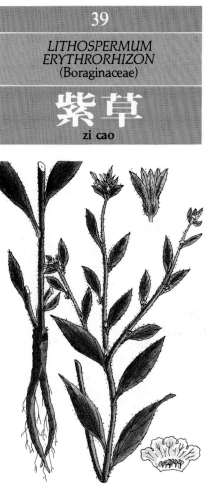

Natural distribution: Northern China, Japan

Parts used: Roots

Nature: Sweet; cold

Affinity: Heart, liver

Effects: Antipyretic; "cools" the blood; antidote to body toxins induced by heat excess

Indications: Heat-rash, itchy skin, etc. due to internal heat excess; measles

Dosage: 5-8 g

Remarks: The drug is applied as an external emollient to eczema, abscesses, and burns; the oil is effective for diaper rash

40

RHINOCEROS UNICORNIS
(Rhinocerotidae)

RHINO HORN

犀角

xi jiao

Natural distribution: Africa, India

Parts used: Horn

Nature: Bitter, sour and salty; cold

Affinity: Heart, liver, stomach

Effects: Antipyretic; cardiotonic; antispasmodic; hemostatic; antidote

Indications: Persistent and serious symptoms of internal heat excess: nosebleed, blood in sputum, dizziness, delirium, convulsions, heat rash, painful dark and scanty urine

Dosage: 1-2 g

Remarks: This drug is very expensive today; water-buffalo horn is often substituted, though it is not as potent and requires larger doses (10g)

41	42	43

41

BOS TAURUS DOMESTICUS or
BUBALUS BUBALIS
(Bovidae)

GALL STONES FROM COW or
WATER-BUFFALO

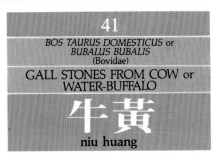

牛黃

niu huang

Natural distribution: Common world-wide
Parts used: Bezoar
Nature: Bitter and sweet; cool
Affinity: Heart, liver
Effects: Antipyretic; diuretic; cardiotonic; sedative; antispasmodic; antidote
Indications: Body heat, irritability, and delirium due to internal heat excess; spasms; sore, swollen, or infected throat; abscesses and sores of heat excess
Dosage: 0.2-0.4 g
Remarks: The genuine item is hard to find and very expensive; substitutes refined from the extract of cow's or pig's gall bladder fluid are common and also quite effective

42

PAEONIA MOUTAN
(Ranunculaceae)

TREE PEONY

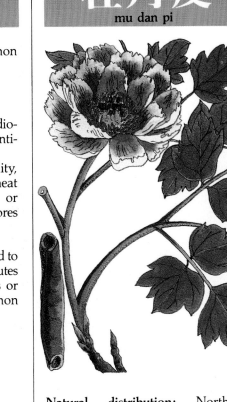

牡丹皮

mu dan pi

Natural distribution: Northern China
Parts used: Skin of the roots
Nature: Pungent and bitter; slightly cold
Affinity: Heart, liver, kidneys
Effects: Antipyretic; "cools" the blood; promotes circulation; anticoagulant; emmenagogue; antiseptic; diuretic
Indications: All symptoms of heat excess: blood in sputum and urine, nosebleeds, irritability, and others; yin-deficiency due to heat excess damage; amenorrhoea; ulcers; infections in intestinal tract
Dosage: 5-10 g
Remarks: The drug has highly effective antiseptic action against a broad range of germs

43

PAEONIA LACTIFLORA
(Ranunculaceae)

CHINESE WHITE PEONY

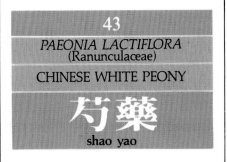

芍藥

shao yao

Natural distribution: China, Manchuria, Siberia, Japan
Parts used: Roots
Nature: Bitter; slightly cold
Affinity: Liver
Effects: Antipyretic; hemostatic; antiseptic; emmenagogue
Indications: All symptoms of heat excess; heat rash; amenorrhoea; ulcers; intestinal infections
Dosage: 5-10 g
Remarks: Two varieties are distinguished: white and red; white variety is tonic to blood and yin-energy; red variety is hemostatic and promotes circulation

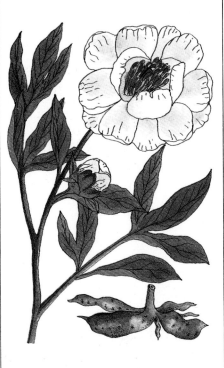

44

ISATIS TINCTORIA
(Crucifereae)

WOAD

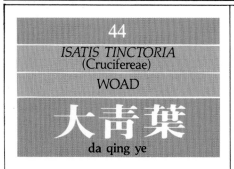

大青葉

da qing ye

Natural distribution: China, Japan
Parts used: Leaves
Nature: Bitter; very cold
Affinity: Heart, stomach
Effects: Antipyretic; antiphlogistic; antidote; antiseptic
Indications: Delirium, fainting spells, heat rash, dry and sore throat, abscesses, and swelling due to internal heat excess; erysipelas
Dosage: 7-15 g
Remarks: Effective preventive in chronic encephalitis; suppresses or kills a broad range of germs

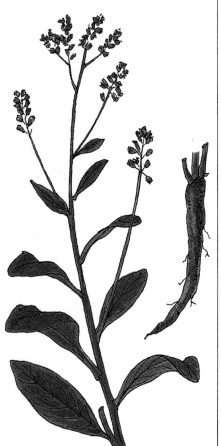

45

SCROPHULARIA NINGPOENSIS
(Scrohpulariaceae)

xuan shen

玄參

xuan shen

Natural distribution: Northern China, Japan
Parts used: Roots
Nature: Bitter and salty; cold
Affinity: Lungs, stomach, kidneys
Effects: Antipyretic, antiphlogistic; refrigerant; tonic to yin-energy; antidote
Indications: All heat excess symptoms: delirium, insomnia, red sore and swollen eyes, abscesses and carbuncles, thirst, inflamed tongue, etc.; laryngitis; tonsillitis
Dosage: 7-10 g
Remarks: Small doses are cardiotonic; large doses impede cardiac functions; the drug also lowers blood sugar

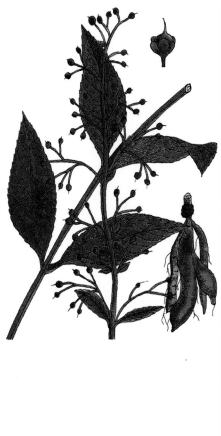

46

IMPERATA CYLINDRICA
(Gramineae)

WOOLLY GRASS

白茅根

bai mao gen

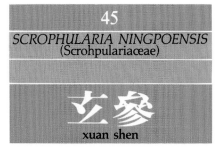

Natural distribution: South China, India, Sri Lanka, Indochina, Africa
Parts used: Roots
Nature: Sweet; cold
Affinity: Lungs, stomach
Effects: Antipyretic; diuretic; demulcent; hemostatic
Indications: All symptoms of heat excess; nausea or vomiting due to dry stomach; cough due to dry lungs; blood in sputum and urine
Dosage: 10-35 g
Remarks: Strong hemostatic action; promotes immediate coagulation in bleeding wounds; suppresses bruising and other forms of internal bleeding

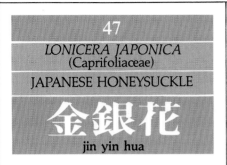

47

LONICERA JAPONICA
(Caprifoliaceae)

JAPANESE HONEYSUCKLE

金銀花

jin yin hua

Natural distribution: China, Japan, Korea
Parts used: Flowers
Nature: Sweet; cold
Affinity: Lungs, stomach, heart, spleen
Effects: Antipyretic; antidote; refrigerant
Indications: Heat-injury moving from external to internal areas: sore, inflamed and swollen throat, blood in stool and sputum; ulcers
Dosage: 10-17 g
Remarks: The entire plant is used in medicine; and infusion of the fresh flowers is applied externally to skin sores and infections

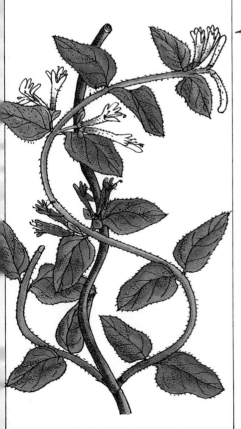

48

FORSYTHIA SUSPENSA
(Oleaceae)

WEEPING GOLDEN BELL

連翹

lian qiao

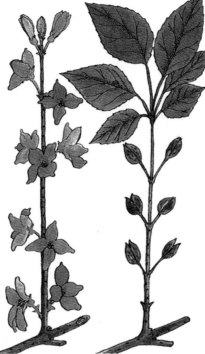

Natural distribution: Northern China, Japan
Parts used: Fruit
Nature: Bitter; slightly cold
Affinity: Heart, gall bladder
Effects: Antipyretic; antidote; antiphlogistic
Indications: Heat-injury moving from external to internal areas: excess body heat, thirst, irritability, heat rash; swelling of lymph glands; erysipelas; breast tumors
Dosage: 5-10 g
Remarks: Similar action as *Lonicera japonica*; used in combination, their efficacy is greatly enhanced

49

TARAXACUM OFFICINALE
(Compositae)

DANDELION

蒲公英

pu gong ying

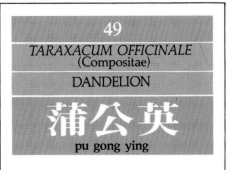

Natural distribution: Temperate zones of the world
Parts used: Whole plant
Nature: Bitter and sweet; cold
Affinity: Liver, stomach
Effects: Antipyretic; antidote; reduces swelling
Indications: Breast tumors; abscesses; tumors and clots in lungs
Dosage: 10-30 g
Remarks: The juice squeezed from the fresh plants is applied directly to poisonous snake-bites as antidote

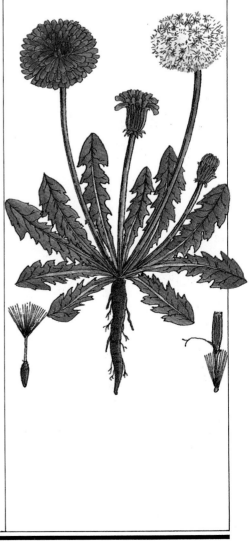

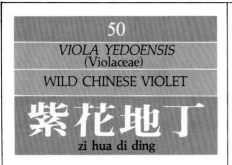

50	51	52
VIOLA YEDOENSIS (Violaceae)	*BELAMCANDA CHINENSIS* (Iridaceae)	*SOPHORA SUBPROSTRATA* (Leguminosae)
WILD CHINESE VIOLET	BLACKBERRY LILY, LEOPARD FLOWER	PIGEON PEA
紫花地丁	射干	廣豆根
zi hua di ding	she gan	guang dou gen

Natural distribution: China, Indochina, Japan, India

Parts used: Whole plant

Nature: Bitter and pungent; cold

Affinity: Heart, liver

Effects: Antipyretic; antidote; antiphlogistic

Indications: Abscesses; carbuncles; boils; ulcers

Dosage: 5-10 g

Remarks: Juice of the fresh root is applied externally to abscesses; juice of the fresh whole plant is applied directly to poisonous snake-bites as antidote

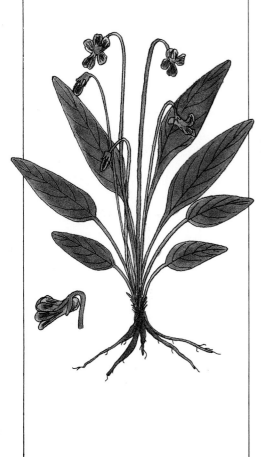

Natural distribution: Southern China, Japan, Korea, Vietnam, Laos

Parts used: Rhizomes and stems

Nature: Bitter; cold

Affinity: Lungs, liver

Effects: Antipyretic; antidote, expectorant; antiphlogistic to upper respiratory tract

Indications: Upper respiratory inflammations; excess phlegm, sputum due to asthma or bronchitis; coughs

Dosage: 3-6 g

Remarks: Slightly poisonous

Natural distribution: Southern China, Indochina, India

Parts used: Roots

Nature: Bitter; cold

Affinity: Heart, lungs

Effects: Antipyretic; antidote; antiphlogistic to respiratory tract

Indications: Throat inflammations and infections

Dosage: 3-8 g

Remarks: Excellent antidote for natural internal toxins produced in body due to heat excess

53

LYCOPERDON PERLATUM
(Lycoperdaceae)

PUFF BALL

馬勃

ma bo

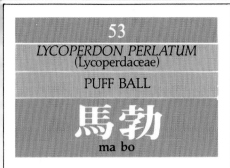

Natural distribution: Common world-wide
Parts used: Spore dust
Nature: Pungent; neutral
Affinity: Lungs
Effects: Antipyretic; antidote; antiphlogistic to respiratory tract; antitussive; hemostatic
Indications: Respiratory problems due to extreme heat excess; excess heat in lungs
Dosage: 1-2 g
Remarks: This drug is also applied externally to bleeding wounds to promote coagulation

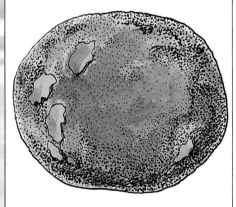

54

CANARIUM ALBUM
(Burseraceae)

CHINESE OLIVE

橄欖

gan lan

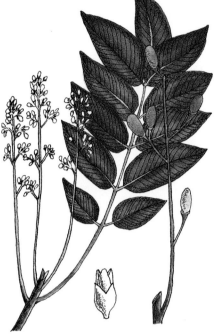

Natural distribution: Southeastern China, Indochina
Parts used: Fruits
Nature: Sweet and sour; neutral
Affinity: Lungs, stomach
Effects: Antipyretic; antidote; antiphlogistic; astringent
Indications: All symptoms of heat excess in stomach and lungs; pharyngitis
Dosage: 5-10 g
Remarks: The fruits are slowly chewed and swallowed to dissolve fish-bones lodged in the throat; the drug is a good antidote for seafood poisoning and allergic reactions

55

PULSATILLA CHINENSIS
(Ranunculaceae)

CHINESE ANEMONE

白頭翁

bai tou weng

Natural distribution: Northern China, Japan, Korea
Parts used: Roots
Nature: Bitter; cold
Affinity: Stomach, large intestine
Effects: Antipyretic; antidote; refrigerant; antidysenteric
Indications: Amoebic dysentery
Dosage: 5-10 g
Remarks: One of the most effective of all drugs for amoebic dysentery; can be used singly in decoction

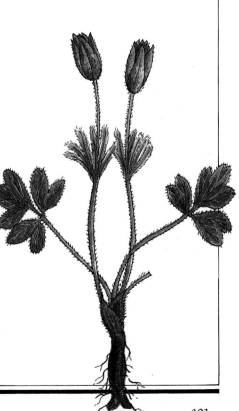

56	57	58
PORTULACA OLERACEA (Portulacaceae) PURSLANE	*BRUCEA JAVANICA* (Simaroubaceae)	*SCUTELLARIA BARBATA* (Labiatae)

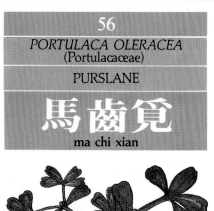

馬齒莧

ma chi xian

鴉胆子

ya dan zi

半枝蓮

ban zhi lian

Natural distribution: Southern China, India, Sumatra
Parts used: Fruits
Nature: Bitter; cold
Affinity: Large intestine
Effects: Antidysenteric; anthelmintic; antipyretic
Indications: Chronic amoebic dysentery; intermittent dysentery; malaria; corns
Dosage: Malaria—7-12 fruits 3 times a day for 5-7 days; dysentery—10-15 fruits 3 times a day for 7 days
Remarks: The drug has strong antiseptic action against amoebic and malarial germs, intestinal parasites, and vaginal infections

Natural distribution: China, Japan
Parts used: Whole plant
Nature: Bitter; cold
Affinity: (Affinity not determined)
Effects: Antipyretic; antidote; diuretic; hemostatic; reduces swellings
Indications: Abscesses and boils due to heat excess; poisonous snake-bites; ulcers in stomach and lungs; cancer in lungs, stomach and intestines
Dosage: 10-30 g
Remarks: This herb was discovered after Li Shizhen's time (Ming); its natural affinities have not been determined; it has been found effective in treating certain forms of cancer

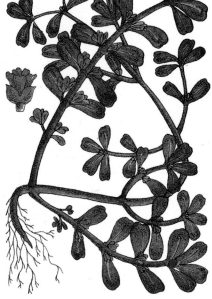

Natural distribution: China, Europe, North America
Parts used: Whole plant
Nature: Sour; cold
Affinity: Liver, large intestine
Effects: Antipyretic; antidote; refrigerant; antidysenteric; antiphlogistic
Indications: Amoebic dysentery; hemorrhoids; abscesses due to heat excess
Dosage: 10-30 g
Remarks: The Chinese eat this plant as a vegetable; may be used safely in high dosages; the fresh herb is best for all therapeutic purposes

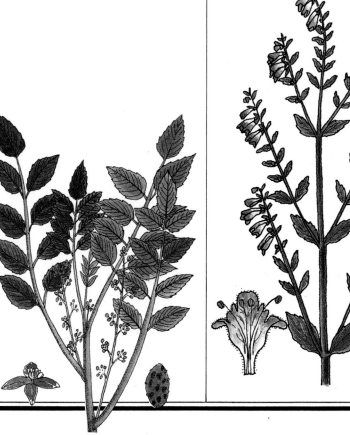

59	60	61
COPTIS SINENSIS (Ranunculaceae)	*SCUTELLARIA BAICALENSIS* (Labiatae)	*PHELLODENDRON AMURENSE* (Rutaceae)
MISHMI BITTER	BAICAL SKULLCAP	SIBERIAN CORK TREE
黄連 **huang lian**	黄芩 **huang qin**	黄柏 **huang bo**

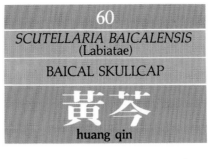

60 — SCUTELLARIA BAICALENSIS

Natural distribution: Northern China, Manchuria, Siberia
Parts used: Roots
Nature: Bitter; cold
Affinity: Heart, lungs, gall bladder, large intestine, small intestine
Effects: Antipyretic; antidote; refrigerant; drying; sedative to restless foetus
Indications: Ailments of "full" and "hot" excess: oppression in chest, thirst with no desire for water, dysentery and diarrhoea, jaundice, body heat, irritability, blood in stool and sputum, nosebleeds
Dosage: 5-8 g
Remarks: The drug also lowers blood pressure, has sedative effects on the central nervous system, and is antiseptic against a broad range of germs

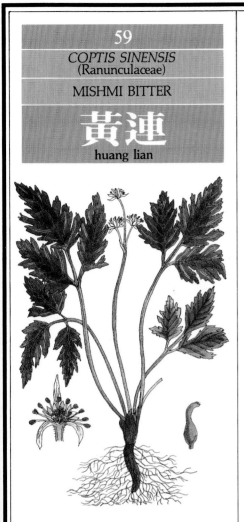

59 — COPTIS SINENSIS

Natural distribution: Central China, northern India
Parts used: Rhizomes
Nature: Bitter; cold
Affinity: Heart, liver, stomach, large intestine
Effects: Antipyretic; drying; antidote; refrigerant
Indications: Ailments of "full" and "hot" excess: oppression in chest, jaundice, dysentery and diarrhoea, abscesses, heat stroke, nosebleeds
Dosage: 3-5 g
Remarks: Juice of the fresh root is used as eye wash for sore, red and swollen eyes and as gargle for abscesses in mouth; strong suppressive action against broad range of germs and toxins

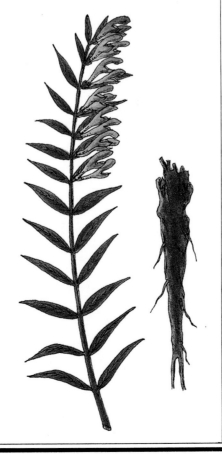

61 — PHELLODENDRON AMURENSE

Natural distribution: Northern China, Japan, Siberia
Parts used: Bark
Nature: Bitter; cold
Affinity: Kidneys, bladder, large intestine
Effects: Antipyretic: drying, refrigerant; antidote
Indications: Ailments of "damp-heat" excess: diarrhoea, jaundice, painful urination, dark leukorrhoea, vaginal swelling and pain, arthritic and rheumatic pain; skin diseases; yin-deficiency; nocturnal emissions
Dosage: 5 g
Remarks: Strong antiseptic action in dysentery, enteritis, cystitis, urethritis; also lowers blood pressure and blood sugar

62	63	64

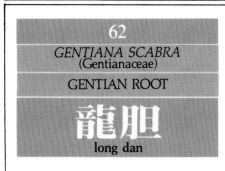

62

GENTIANA SCABRA
(Gentianaceae)

GENTIAN ROOT

龍胆

long dan

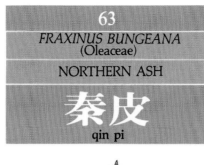

63

FRAXINUS BUNGEANA
(Oleaceae)

NORTHERN ASH

秦皮

qin pi

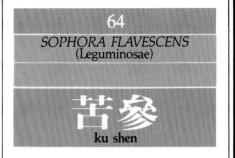

64

SOPHORA FLAVESCENS
(Leguminosae)

苦參

ku shen

Natural distribution: China
Parts used: Roots
Nature: Bitter; cold
Affinity: Liver, gall bladder
Effects: Antipyretic; drying; refrigerant; stomachic
Indications: "Damp-heat" excess ailments: jaundice, dark leukorrhoea, pain and swelling in scrotum, headaches, sore eyes, chest pains; tantrums in children
Dosage: 3-8 g
Remarks: Taken in small doses half an hour before meals, the drug promotes digestion by inducing secretion of digestive juices in stomach; taken after meals, it will impair flow of digestive juices and impede digestion

Natural distribution: China
Parts used: Roots
Nature: Bitter; cold
Affinity: Heart, liver, large intestine, small intestine, stomach
Effects: Antipyretic; drying, anthelmintic
Indications: "Damp-heat" ailments: dysentery and diarrhoea, jaundice, leukorrhoea, vaginal infections, sores and itchy skin, allergic reactions; leprosy
Dosage: 4-7 g
Remarks: Used internally and externally, the drug is an excellent remedy for sores, pruritus and other skin ailments

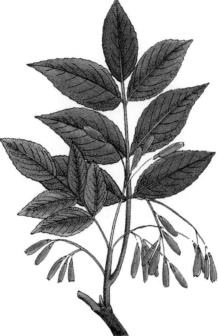

Natural distribution: Northern China
Parts used: Bark
Nature: Bitter and sour; cold
Affinity: Liver, gall bladder, large intestine
Effects: Antipyretic; drying; promotes vision
Indications: Dysentery; painful bowel movements; swollen, aching and red eyes
Dosage: 5-8 g
Remarks: A decoction of this herb is used as antiphlogistic eye wash

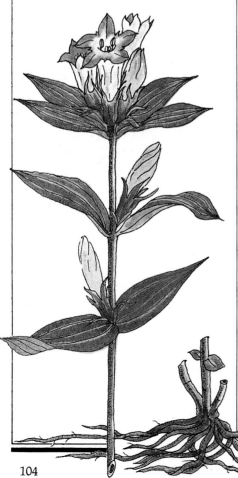

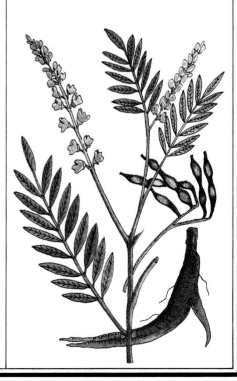

LYCIUM CHINENSE
(Solanaceae)
CHINESE WOLFBERRY,
BOX THORN

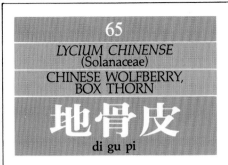

地骨皮

di gu pi

Natural distribution: China, Japan
Parts used: Skin of the roots
Nature: Sweet and plain; cold
Affinity: Lungs, kidneys
Effects: Antipyretic; refrigerant; antitussive
Indications: Ailments of heat excess in lungs: asthma, coughs, blood in sputum; blood in urine; body heat, fevers due to yin-deficiency
Dosage: 10-15 g
Remarks: The fresh root lowers blood pressure and blood sugar

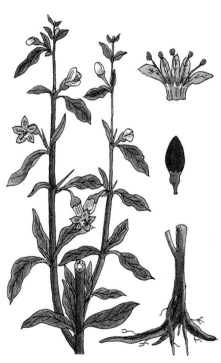

66

ARTEMISIA ANNUA
(Compositae)
SWEET WORMWOOD

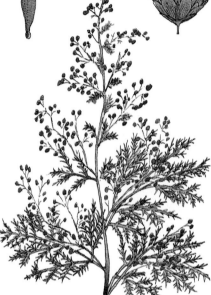

黄花蒿

huang hua hao

Natural distribution: China, Vietnam, Siberia, India
Parts used: Stems and leaves
Nature: Bitter; cold
Affinity: Liver, gall bladder
Effects: Antipyretic
Indications: Summer colds; sweatless fevers; malaria; nocturnal sweats; heat excess
Dosage: 5-10 g
Remarks: An excellent refrigerant remedy in ailments of "empty-hot" excess

---

CYNANCHUM ATRATUM
(Asclepiadaceae)

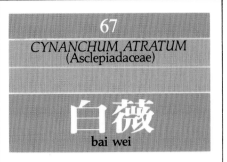

白薇

bai wei

Natural distribution: Northern China, Japan
Parts used: Roots
Nature: Bitter and salty; cold
Affinity: Liver, stomach
Effects: Antipyretic; refrigerant to blood; diuretic
Indications: Extreme and prolonged ailments of heat excess: coughs due to excess heat in lungs; heat excess due to yin-deficiency; painful, hot, and scanty urine
Dosage: 4-7 g

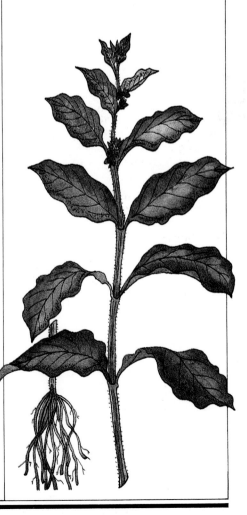

AROMATIC DEHYDRATORS OR "TRANSFORM MOISTURE"

Drugs which are aromatic and tend to drive out or convert excess moisture in the body fall under this category. The spleen is the organ most sensitive to damp excess, which impedes its digestive and distributive functions. Therefore, these herbs are also called "spleen restoratives."

They are employed against sluggish stagnation of blood and energy, impeded spleen function and other damp excess ailments. Common symptoms of such ailments are oppressive sensations in the chest, vomiting bile, loose bowels, lack of appetite, fatigue, a sweet taste in the mouth, profuse saliva, or white and slippery tongue fur. Injuries of "damp heat" and "damp summer heat," such as excess phlegm in the respiratory tract, are also remedied with these herbs.

Most of the drugs in this category are "pungent" and "warm" in nature. They are all aromatics which tend to dehydrate the system and thus have adverse effects on yin-energy and fluid balance. Patients with yin-deficiency, fluid-deficiency, or *qi*-deficiency should use them with caution.

AGASTACHE RUGOSA
(Labiatae)

HYSSOP

藿香
huo xiang

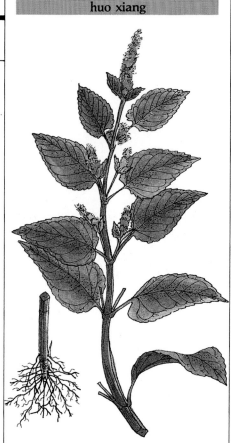

Natural distribution: China, Japan, Vietnam, Laos
Parts used: Leaves and stems
Nature: Pungent and sweet; slightly warm
Affinity: Spleen, stomach, lungs
Effects: Drying, stomachic; carminative; diaphoretic
Indications: Damp excess in stomach and spleen: oppression in chest, nausea and vomiting, diarrhoea; sluggishness and oppression due to "damp summer heat" excess; external injuries of "wind-cold"
Dosage: 5-7 g
Remarks: A highly effective preventive for heat stroke and summer colds

---

EUPATORIUM FORTUNEI
(Compositae)

佩蘭
pei lan

Natural distribution: China, Japan
Parts used: Stems and leaves
Nature: Pungent; neutral
Affinity: Spleen, stomach
Effects: Drying; stomachic; antipyretic; diaphoretic
Indications: Ailments of damp excess in spleen and stomach: dyspepsia, oppression in chest, nausea and vomiting, diarrhoea, pressure and pain in abdomen; summer chills
Dosage: 3-10 g
Remarks: A highly effective preventive remedy for heat stroke and summer colds when mixed with *Agastache rugosa*

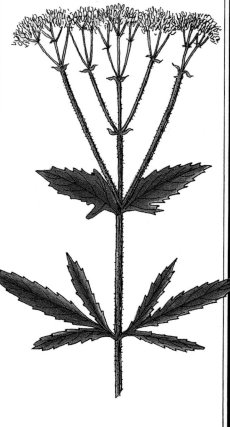

70	71	72
ATRACTYLODES CHINENSIS (Compositae) THISTLE TYPE	*MAGNOLIA OFFICINALIS* (Magnoliaceae) MAGNOLIA	*AMOMUM XANTHIOIDES* (Zingiberaceae) GRAINS-OF-PARADISE
蒼朮 cang zhu	厚朴 hou po	砂仁 sha ren

Natural distribution: China, Japan, Korea
Parts used: Roots
Nature: Bitter; warm
Affinity: Spleen, stomach
Effects: Drying; stomachic; eliminates "wind-damp" symptoms
Indications: Ailments of damp excess in spleen and stomach: diarrhoea, nausea and vomiting, oppression in chest and abdomen, leukorrhoea, gastronenteritis; "damp-heat" injuries: aching joints and muscles, swelling and pain in feet and legs, weakness and sluggishness
Dosage: 5-10 g
Remarks: Effective remedy for night blindness

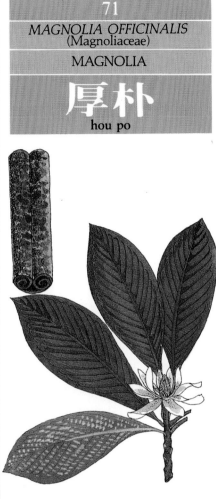

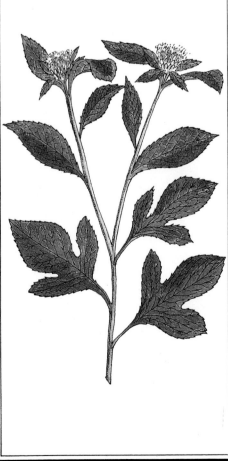

Natural distribution: Central China
Parts used: Bark
Nature: Bitter and pungent: warm
Affinity: Spleen, stomach, lungs, large intestine
Effects: Drying; digestive; antiemetic
Indications: Ailments of damp excess in spleen and stomach: abdominal pressure and pain, oppression in chest, excess phlegm in respiratory tract, shortness of breath
Dosage: 6-10 g
Remarks: Especially effective in relieving pressure, fullness and oppression in abdominal region

Natural distribution: Southern China, Indochina
Parts used: Seeds
Nature: Pungent; warm
Affinity: Spleen, stomach, kidneys
Effects: Drying; stomachic; digestive; carminative; decongestant; sedative to restless foetus
Indications: Damp excess in spleen and stomach: oppression in chest and abdomen, diarrhoea, dyspepsia; nausea and vomiting during pregnancy; restless foetus
Dosage: 2-4 g

DIURETIC OR "PASS WATER, FACILITATE URINE"

Herbs whose primary pharmacodynamic effects are to eliminate excess water from the system by converting it to urine and facilitating its passage through the bladder and ureter are called "diuretics." These drugs all increase the quantity of urine and frequency of urination. They are mostly of "sweet" and "plain" flavour and "neutral" energy. Diuretic herbs are used against all symptoms of water retention, "damp-heat," and "damp-cold" ailments. Common symptoms are difficult and/or painful urination, murky urine, painful joints and sinews, jaundice, sore and rashes on skin, excess phlegm, swelling and leukorrhoea.

Diuretics should be sparingly used by patients suffering from yin-deficiency or fluid deficiency.

73
PORIA COCOS (Polyporaceae)
SUBTERRANEAN FUNGUS
(known as TUCKAHOE, INDIAN BREAD, VIRGINIA TRUFFLE)

73
PORIA COCOS (Polyporaceae)
SUBTERRANEAN FUNGUS
(known as TUCKAHOE, INDIAN BREAD, VIRGINIA TRUFFLE)

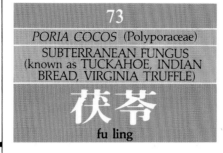

伏苓
fu ling

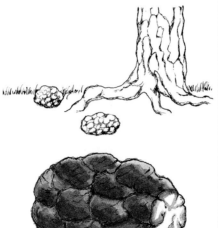

Natural distribution: Common world-wide
Parts used: Fungal body
Nature: Sweet; neutral
Affinity: Heart, lungs, spleen, stomach, kidneys
Effects: Diuretic; stomachic; digestive; sedative
Indications: Difficult urination; swelling; oppression in abdomen; lack of appetite; diarrhoea; excess phlegm; coughing; insomnia; nervousness; heart palpitations
Dosage: 5-10 g

74
ALISMA PLANTAGO-AQUATICA (Alismataceae)
WATER PLANTAIN

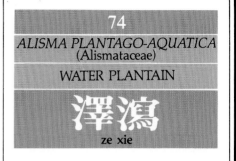

澤瀉
ze xie

Natural distribution: Northern China, northern Europe, North America
Parts used: Tubers
Nature: Sweet; cold
Affinity: Kidneys, bladder
Effects: Diuretic; refrigerant
Indications: Difficult urination; swelling; diarrhoea; murky urine; leukorrhoea; excess phlegm
Dosage: 5-15 g
Remarks: Strong affinity for the female genitalia

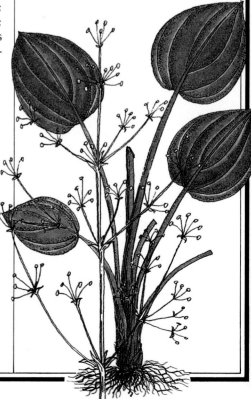

車前子

che qian zi

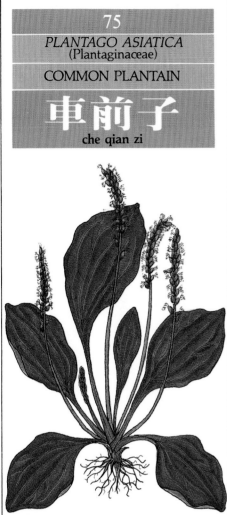

Natural distribution: Common world-wide
Parts used: Seeds
Nature: Sweet; cold
Affinity: Liver, kidneys, small intestine, lungs
Effects: Diuretic; antidysenteric; expectorant; improves vision
Indications: Difficult or painful urination; diarrhoea of "full-hot" type; aching and swollen eyes; blurry vision; coughs; excess phlegm
Dosage: 5-10 g
Remarks: This is the only diuretic that also tonifies the kidneys and appears in many aphrodisiac prescriptions; it also lowers blood pressure

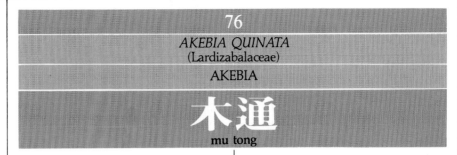

木通

mu tong

Natural distribution: Eastern China, Japan
Parts used: Stems
Nature: Bitter; cold
Affinity: Heart, lungs, small intestine, bladder
Effects: Diuretic; antiphlogistic; promotes lactation

Indications: Abscesses on tongue and mouth; insomnia; restlessness; dark and scanty urine; difficult and painful urination; pain and swelling in feet and legs; insufficient lactation
Dosage: 4-7 g
Remarks: The drug brewed together with pork knuckles is highly effective in promoting lactation; doses should not exceed 15 g a day

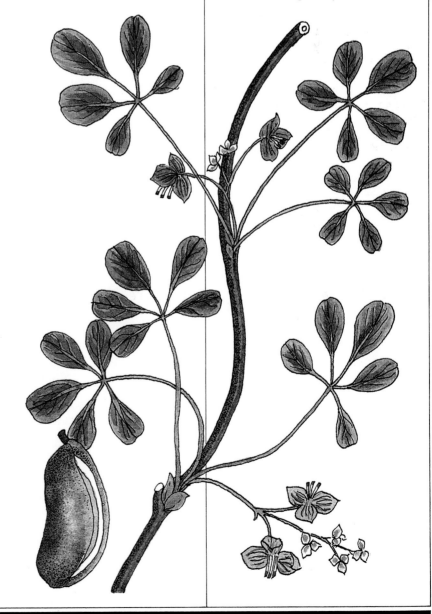

77	78	79
ARTEMISIA CAPILLARIS (Compositae)	*COIX LACRYMA-JOBI* (Gramineae)	*ZEA MAYS* (Gramineae)
CHINESE MOXA WEED	JOB'S TEARS	INDIAN CORN

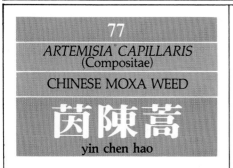

茵陳蒿

yin chen hao

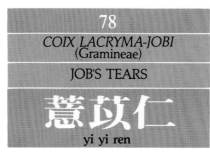

薏苡仁

yi yi ren

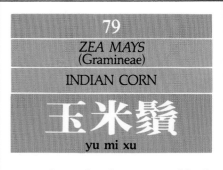

玉米鬚

yu mi xu

Natural distribution: Northern China, Japan, Taiwan
Parts used: Stems and leaves of the young shoots
Nature: Bitter; neutral
Affinity: Spleen, stomach, liver, gall bladder
Effects: Diuretic; antipyretic
Indications: Jaundice due to "damp-heat" excess
Dosage: 10-15 g
Remarks: Effective remedy for jaundice; the drug also promotes secretion of bile when insufficient

Natural distribution: China, India, Africa, America
Parts used: Seeds
Nature: Sweet and plain; slightly cold
Affinity: Spleen, stomach, lungs
Effects: Diuretic; decongestant to lungs; digestive; refrigerant; anti-dysenteric
Indications: Dark and scanty urine; swelling; painful joints, sinews and bones due to damp excess; ulcers in the stomach or lungs; diarrhoea and dyspepsia due to damp injury to spleen
Dosage: 10-30 g
Remarks: This is a common food item in China and Japan and contains 17 percent protein; the drug tonifies yang-energy; a liquor fermented from the seeds is effective in relieving rheumatic pains

Natural distribution: North America, China
Parts used: The pistils and stamens of the young flowers; the "corn-silk" of the mature ears
Nature: Sweet; neutral (affinity not determined; the herb was introduced to China from North America after Li Shizhen's time)
Effects: Diuretic; reduces swelling
Indications: Difficult and painful urination; swelling jaundice due to damp excess; liver inflammations
Dosage: 15-30 g
Remarks: Research has shown this herb to be highly effective in dissolving gall stones; it also lowers blood pressure and blood sugar

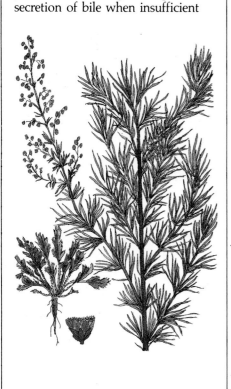

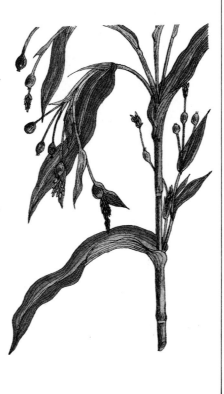

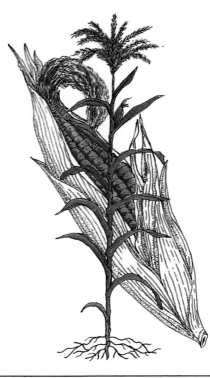

80

DIOSCOREA HYPOGLAUCA
(Dioscoreaceae)

LONG YAM

萆薢

bei xie

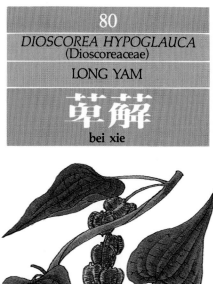

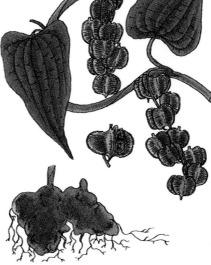

Natural distribution: Sichuan, Henan, Hubei
Parts used: Roots
Nature: Bitter; neutral
Affinity: Liver, stomach
Effects: Diuretic; eliminates "wind-damp" symptoms
Indications: Murky urine; urethritis; leukorrhoea; pains due to "wind-damp" injury: stiff joints, sore muscles, pain and stiffness in lower back and knees
Dosage: 10-15 g

81

HYDROUS MAGNESIUM SILICATE

TALC

滑石

hua shi

Natural distribution: Common mineral
Parts used: Powder
Nature: Sweet; cold
Affinity: Stomach, bladder
Effects: Diuretic; antiphlogistic; refrigerant
Indications: Difficult urination; urethritis; diarrhoea due to "damp-heat;" summer fevers and chills; oppression in chest
Dosage: 5-10 g
Remarks: Applied externally, it has a drying effect on surface moisture; effective remedy for boils and prickly heat

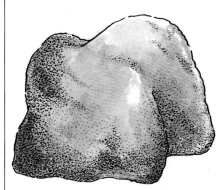

82

MALVA VERTICILLATA
(Malvaceae)

FARMERS' TOBACCO

冬葵子

dong kui zi

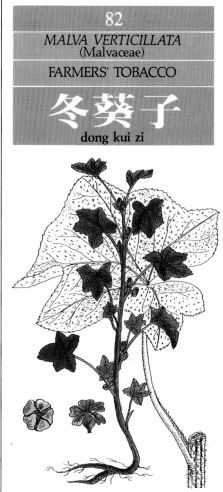

Natural distribution: Southern China, Indochina
Parts used: Seeds
Nature: Sweet; cold
Affinity: Large intestine, small intestine
Effects: Diuretic; promotes lactation
Indications: Difficult urination; urethritis; swelling; insufficient lactation; swollen and painful breasts
Dosage: 5-15 g
Remarks: Promotes lactation and facilitates secretion in breast-feeding mothers

111

ANTIRHEUMATIC OR "EXPEL WIND-DAMP"

Herbs which expel "evil" wind-and-damp-excess from the body and thereby relieve painful symptoms of rheumatism and arthritis in joints, sinews, muscles, bones and meridians belong in the "antirheumatic" group. Their primary pharmacodynamic effects are to drive out "wind-damp" excess accumulated in the body and to facilitate the flow of energy in the meridians. There are many forms of this ailment, and the mix of drugs used in antirheumatic prescriptions must follow detailed differential diagnosis.

If the ailment is external, they are mixed with diaphoretic drugs. If "wind-damp" injury has moved into the meridians and joints, causing energy and blood stagnation, they are used with blood regulators and energy regulators. If the ailment combines with heat excess and its attendant symptoms, these herbs are mixed with antipyretic, refrigerant drugs. If the patient suffers from energy and/or blood deficiency, these herbs should be used along with herbs which tonify and nourish energy and blood.

83
ANGELICA PUBESCENS
(Umbelliferae)

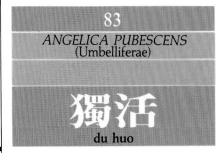

獨活
du huo

Natural distribution: Sichuan, Hubei
Parts used: Roots
Nature: Pungent and bitter; slightly warm
Affinity: Kidneys, bladder
Effects: Antirheumatic; analgesic
Indications: Rheumatism and arthritis; pain and stiffness in lower back and knees
Dosage: 4-10 g

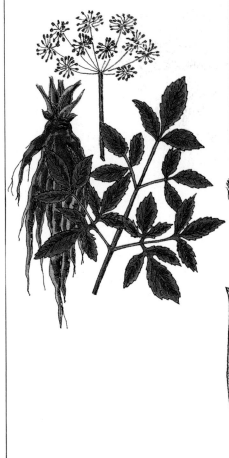

84
CLERODENDRUM TRICHOTOMUM
(Verbenaceae)

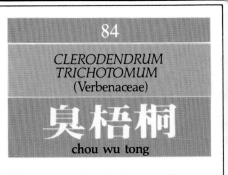

臭梧桐
chou wu tong

Natural distribution: Jiangsu, Shandong, Anhui
Parts used: Tender leaves
Nature: Bitter; cold
Affinity: Liver
Effects: Antirheumatic
Indications: Rheumatism and arthritis; pruritus due to damp excess; high blood pressure; hypertension
Dosage: 10-15 g
Remarks: The drug effectively lowers blood pressure if the tender leaves are picked before the flowers bloom; they should be brewed briefly over low heat; the roots are also used to lower blood pressure

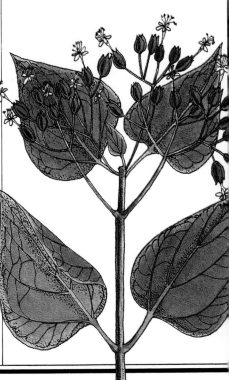

85	86	87
GENTIANA MACROPHYLLA (Gentianaceae)	*CHAENOMELES LAGENARIA* (Rosaceae)	*ELEUTHEROCOCCUS GRACILISTYLUS* (Araliaceae)
GENTIAN	CHINESE QUINCE	ELEUTHEROS
秦艽 qin jiao	木瓜 mu gua	五加皮 wu jia pi

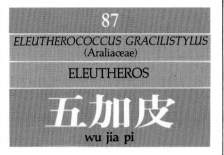

Natural distribution: China, Japan
Parts used: Skin of the roots and stems
Nature: Pungent and bitter; warm
Affinity: Liver, kidneys
Effects: Antirheumatic; analgesic; diuretic; tonifies ligaments and tendons
Indications: Rheumatism and arthritis; cramps; liver and kidney deficiencies; weak lower back and legs
Dosage: 5-10 g
Remarks: A strong liquor made with this herb has effective antirheumatic action and also tonifies general and sexual vitality

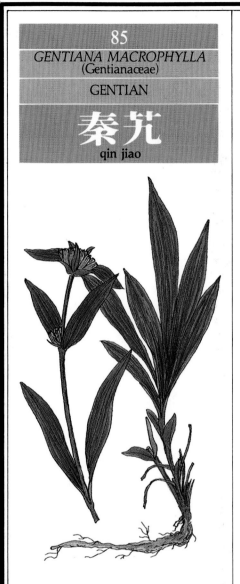

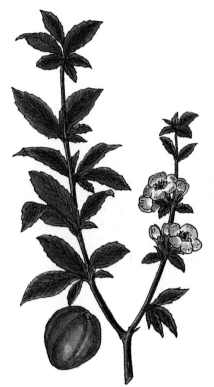

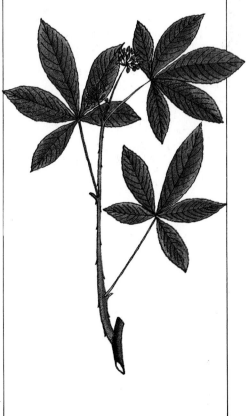

Natural distribution: Yunnan, Sichuan
Parts used: Roots
Nature: Bitter and pungent; neutral
Affinity: Stomach, liver, gall bladder
Effects: Antirheumatic; antipyretic; analgesic
Indications: Rheumatism and arthritis: painful and stiff extremities, tight muscles; jaundice due to "damp-heat" excess; yin-deficiency
Dosage: 4-10 g

Natural distribution: Northern China, India, Taiwan
Parts used: Fruit
Nature: Sour; warm
Affinity: Liver, spleen
Effects: Antirheumatic; antispasmodic; astringent; analgesic; stomachic
Indications: Rheumatism and arthritis; swelling in feet and legs; weak lower back and knees; stomach cramps due to diarrhoea and vomiting; painful legs; spasms
Dosage: 3-10 g
Remarks: Especially effective antispasmodic for cramps in the calves

88

CLEMATIS CHINENSIS
(Ranunculaceae)

CLEMATIS VINE

威靈仙

wei ling xian

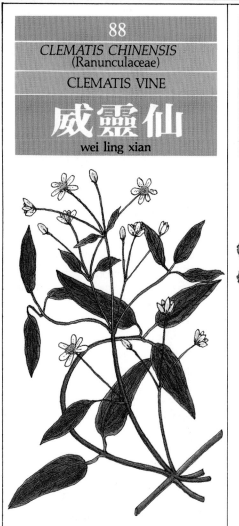

Natural distribution: China, Taiwan, Vietnam
Parts used: Roots
Nature: Pungent; warm
Affinity: Bladder
Effects: Antirheumatic; analgesic; diuretic; antipyretic
Indications: Rhumatism and arthritis
Dosage: 5-10 g
Remarks: 15 g of the drug in decoction with 250 g of rice vinegar dissolves fish bones lodged in the throat; it is incompatible with tea

89

LUFFA CYLINDRICA
(Cucurbitaceae)

A TYPE OF GOURD

絲瓜絡

si gua luo

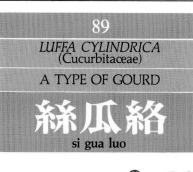

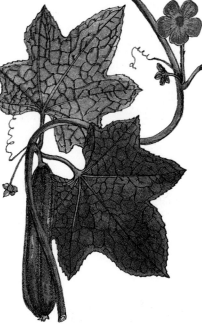

Natural distribution: China, Indochina, Philippines, Japan
Parts used: The fibres of the fully matured fruits
Nature: Sweet; neutral
Affinity: Lungs, stomach, liver
Effects: Antirheumatic; clears the meridians; analgesic; hemostatic
Indications: Rheumatic pains in joints and sinews; aches in chest and rib-cage; painful breast tumours
Dosage: 5-10 g
Remarks: The flesh of the fruit is used as a cooling food item in China

90

AGKISTRODON ACUTUS
(Viperidae)

VIPER SNAKE

白花蛇

bai hua she

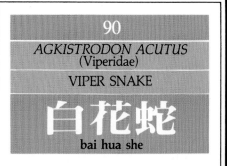

Natural distribution: Eastern China, Southeast Asia
Parts used: The entire body without the head
Nature: Sweet and salty; warm
Affinity: Liver
Effects: Antirheumatic; sedative; anthelmintic
Indications: Rheumatism and arthritis; facial paralysis; paralytic strokes; leprosy; ringworm
Dosage: 4-10 g
Remarks: Poisonous; the drug is highly effective against tetanus infections and attendant spasmic convulsions

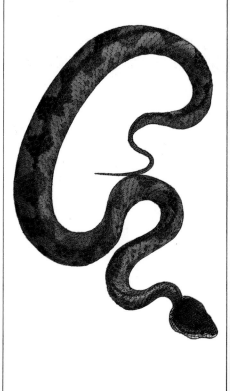

WARMING OR "WARM INTERIOR, DISPEL COLD"

Herbs which warm the interior and dispel cold to correct symptoms of "internal-cold" ailments are called "warming" drugs. Their nature tends towards the warm and hot type. *The Internal Book of Huang-Di* states, "If it's cold, warm it up."

"Internal-cold" ailments are of two kinds: one results from external "evil-cold" invading the interior regions with attendant symptoms of nausea and vomiting, diarrhoea, yang-energy injuries, cold and painful sensations in chest and abdomen, lack of appetite, etc. The other type develops internally when the heart and/or kidneys are "empty" of yang-energy, thereby permitting yin-cold to rise inside, with attendant symptoms of perspiration, fear of cold, cold breath, cold hands and feet and other symptoms of yang-deficiency.

When applying these drugs therapeutically, attention should be paid to the following points:

— In cases of external cold moving
— inward but still displaying certain external symptoms, they should be used together with diaphoretic herbs.
— In hot summer weather or in patients whose bodies are by nature overly "hot," these drugs should be used in smaller doses.
— Warming drugs are generally pungent, warm and dehydrating and should be used with caution in patients with yin-deficiency and fluid deficiency.

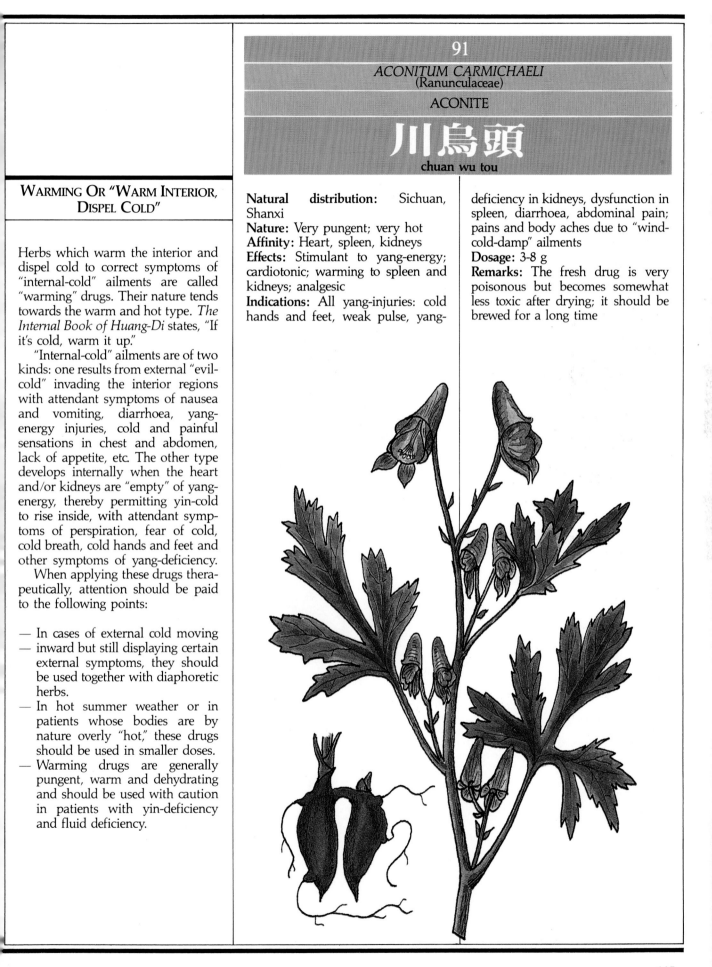

91

ACONITUM CARMICHAELI
(Ranunculaceae)

ACONITE

川烏頭
chuan wu tou

Natural distribution: Sichuan, Shanxi
Nature: Very pungent; very hot
Affinity: Heart, spleen, kidneys
Effects: Stimulant to yang-energy; cardiotonic; warming to spleen and kidneys; analgesic
Indications: All yang-injuries: cold hands and feet, weak pulse, yang-deficiency in kidneys, dysfunction in spleen, diarrhoea, abdominal pain; pains and body aches due to "wind-cold-damp" ailments
Dosage: 3-8 g
Remarks: The fresh drug is very poisonous but becomes somewhat less toxic after drying; it should be brewed for a long time

92

CINNAMOMUM CASSIA
(Lauraceae)

CASSIA, CHINESE CINNAMON

肉桂
rou gui

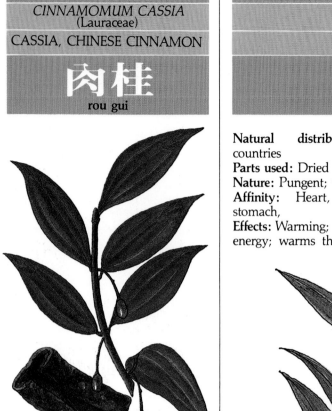

Natural distribution: Southern China, Indochina, Sumatra

Parts used: Unscraped bark of the large trees

Nature: Pungent and sweet; very hot

Affinity: Liver, kidneys, spleen

Effects: Tonic to yang-energy; stimulant; warming; analgesic

Indications: Yang-deficiency in kidneys, yang-deficiency in spleen; cold hands and feet, cold, painful stomach, lack of appetite, diarrhoea; lack of vitality due to prolonged illness; blood and energy deficiency; dysmenorrhoea

Dosage: 1-5 g

Remarks: This medication is pharmacodynamically different from the tender stalks used for diaphoretic purposes

93

ZINGIBER OFFICINALE
(Zingiberaceae)

GINGER

乾薑
gan jiang

Natural distribution: Tropical countries

Parts used: Dried rhizomes

Nature: Pungent; warm

Affinity: Heart, lungs, spleen, stomach, kidneys

Effects: Warming; stimulant to yang-energy; warms the lungs; dissolves phlegm; stomachic; antiemetic

Indications: Cold excess in spleen and stomach: nausea and vomiting, diarrhoea, cold and painful abdomen, cold hands and feet, weak pulse; cold excess in lungs: cough, profuse clear sputum

Dosage: 3-8 g

Remarks: The fresh root is used as a remedy for colds, cold stomach, nausea and seafood poisoning

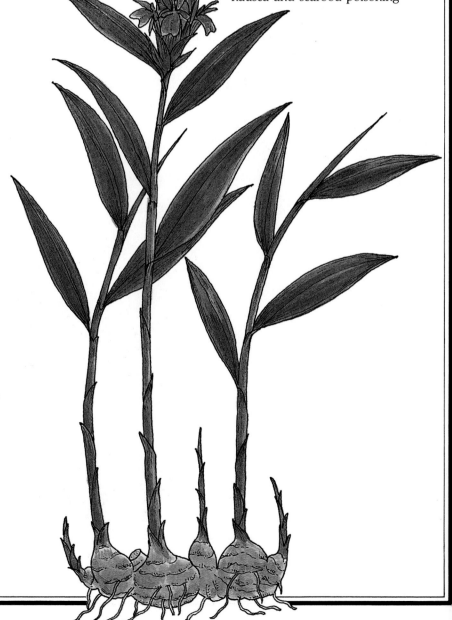

94	95	96
EUODIA RUTAECARPA (Rutaceæ)	*SYZYGIUM AROMATICUM* (Myrtaceæ) CLOVE TREE	*FOENICULUM VULGARE* (Umbelliferae) FENNEL

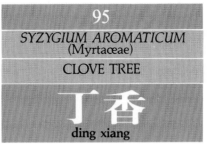

吳茱萸
wu zhu yu

丁香
ding xiang

茴香
hui xiang

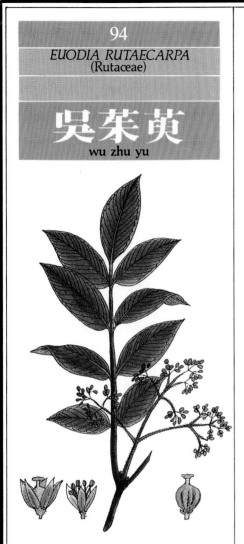

Natural distribution: East Indies, India, West Indies, Brazil
Parts used: Floral buds (cloves)
Nature: Pungent; warm
Affinity: Lungs, stomach, spleen, kidneys
Effects: Warming; antiemetic; stimulant; carminative; tonic to yang-energy; warms the kidneys
Indications: Vomiting and burping; yang-deficiency in kidneys; leukorrhoea
Dosage: 2-5 g
Remarks: This is a common remedy for excessive burping; the oil of the cloves is an excellent local anaesthetic; the drug promotes circulation

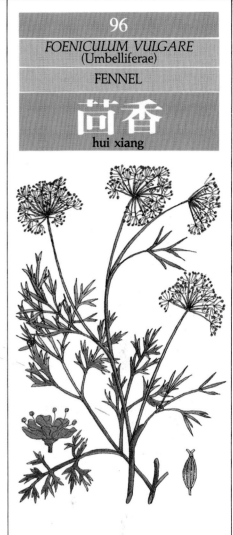

Natural distribution: Southeastern China, Japan, India
Parts used: Fruits
Nature: Pungent and bitter; very hot
Affinity: Liver, stomach, spleen, kidneys
Effects: Warming; analgesic; antiemetic; anthelmintic
Indications: Abdominal pains due to internal-cold; painful rib-cage; pains in scrotum; dysmenorrhoea; dysfunctions of liver and stomach
Dosage: 3-5 g
Remarks: Highly effective anthelmintic against pinworms; tonic to the uterus

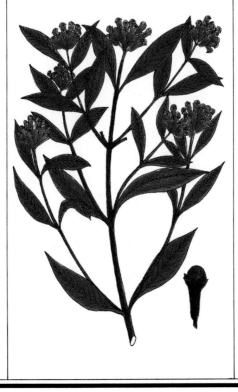

Natural distribution: Asia, Europe, North Africa
Parts used: Fruits
Nature: Pungent; warm
Affinity: Liver, kidneys, spleen, stomach
Effects: Regulates and balances *qi*; analgesic; stomachic; carminative
Indications: Ailments of cold excess: hernias and pains in groin, drooping testicle, pain and cold in abdomen; nausea and vomiting due to cold excess in stomach
Dosage: 2-5 g
Remarks: The drug sometimes causes flatulence and burping

RESUSCITATE, REVIVE OR "OPEN SPIRIT-GATE"

Resuscitive herbs are those which restore consciousness and revive the spirit. They are used in fainting spells, children's convulsions, epilepsy, strokes and other instances of sudden unconsciousness.

Unconsciousness due to heat excess is indicated by flushed complexion, body heat, yellow tongue fur and a rapid pulse. In such cases, resuscitives are combined with "heat-clearing" drugs. Unconsciousness due to cold excess (pale complexion, cold extremities, white tongue fur and slow pulse) is treated in combination with "warming" drugs.

These drugs are generally reserved for use in emergencies: their prolonged use is damaging to the body's primordial energies, *yuan qi*. If patients are weak or display symptoms of profuse, cold sweat, special care should be taken in using these drugs.

97

DRYOBALANOPS AROMATICA
(Dipterocarpaceae)

BORNEO CAMPHOR TREE

龍腦香
long nao xiang

Natural distribution: Malaysia
Parts used: Coagulated resinous fissures of the tree
Nature: Pungent and bitter; slightly cold
Affinity: Heart, spleen, lungs
Effects: Resuscitive; antipyretic; analgesic; antispasmodic

Indications: Fainting; convulsions and spasms; used externally on abscesses, boils, ringworm, cold sores, conjunctivitis, nasal mucositis, coughs
Dosage: 0.18-0.35 g
Remarks: The drug's analgesic and antipyretic properties make it an excellent external remedy for abscesses, boils, sores, sore throat and other external heat excess symptoms

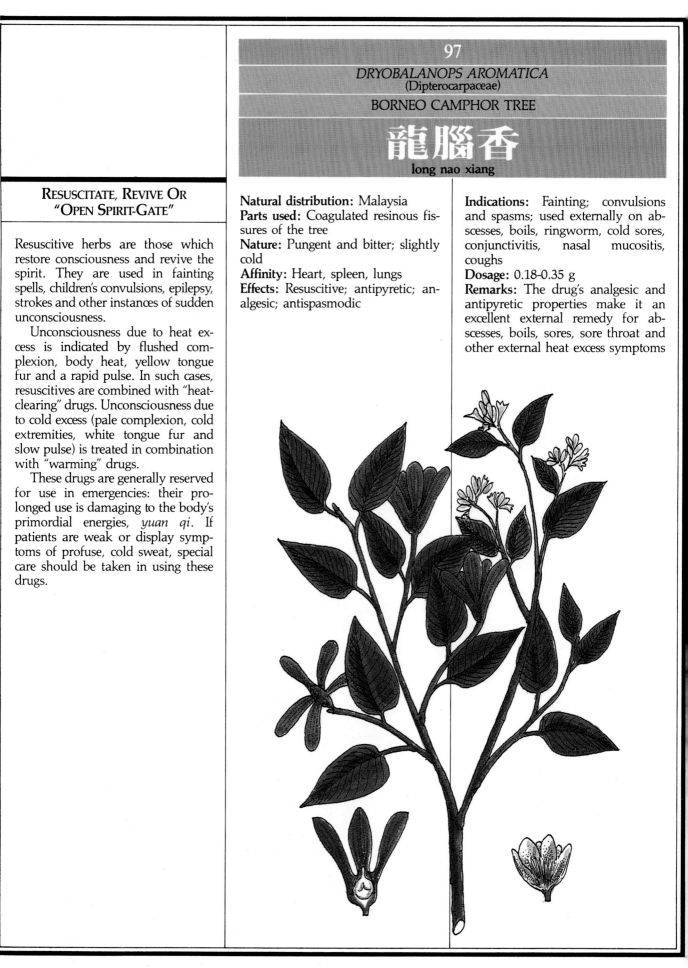

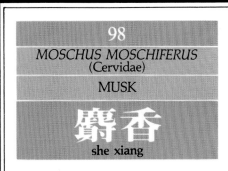

98
MOSCHUS MOSCHIFERUS
(Cervidae)

MUSK

麝香
she xiang

Natural distribution: Tibet, northern India, Siberia
Parts used: Dried secretion of the preputial follicles of the musk-deer
Nature: Pungent; warm
Affinity: Heart, spleen
Effects: Resuscitive; cardiotonic; promotes circulation; stimulant
Indications: Fainting; delirium; semi-conscious states; amenorrhoea; traumatic injuries; retained placenta or foetus
Dosage: 0.2-0.4 g
Remarks: Pregnant women should not be exposed to the drug, for it may induce miscarriage

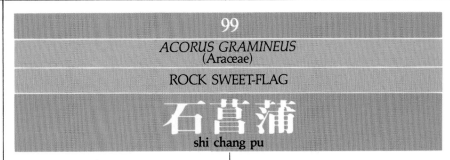

99
ACORUS GRAMINEUS
(Araceae)

ROCK SWEET-FLAG

石菖蒲
shi chang pu

Natural distribution: Southern China, Japan, Tibet, India
Parts used: Rhizomes
Nature: Pungent; warm
Affinity: Heart, liver
Effects: Resuscitive; dissolves phlegm in respiratory tract; stomachic; digestive

Indications: Fainting due to heat excess or excess phlegm; hysteria; ringing in the ears and deafness; oppression in the chest; chronic dysentery
Dosage: Dry 3-8 g; fresh 10-15 g
Remarks: Sedative in insomnia; also a good digestive

119

SEDATIVE OR "CALM THE SPIRIT"

Drugs which calm the nerves, relax the body and quieten the spirit are called "sedatives." They are of two types: one type is derived from heavy minerals and shellfish and is used in cases of over-stimulation and excitement due to "full" ailments. The other type is derived from plants which nourish the heart and tonify the liver. These are used when the symptoms indicate "empty" ailments. Common symptoms for which sedative medications are used include jittery, "floating" yang-energy, insomnia, hysteria, traumatic shock, fright, nervous irritability, quick temper, and other nervous disorders of yang-injury. If symptoms combine with heat excess, "heat-clearing" drugs should be included in the treatment. If symptoms are caused by excess liver-yang ascending, drugs which are specifically sedative to the liver should be combined with regular sedatives. Patients with blood, heart, or liver-yin deficiencies should be treated with sedative drugs which nourish yin-energy and tonify blood.

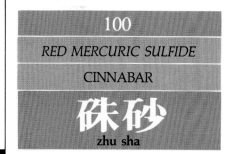

100
RED MERCURIC SULFIDE
CINNABAR

硃砂
zhu sha

Natural distribution: Common mineral
Parts used: Ground powder
Nature: Sweet; slightly cold
Affinity: Heart
Effects: Sedative; antidote; antispasmodic
Indications: Hypertension; nervous excitement; insomnia; traumatic shock; fright; applied externally to abscesses on body, tongue, and mouth, and swollen, painful throat
Dosage: 0.5-1.5 g
Remarks: Slightly poisonous; an effective remedy for chronic nightmares and hysteria; ancient Taoist alchemists attributed great power to this mineral and it was a principal ingredient in their "Elixir of Life"

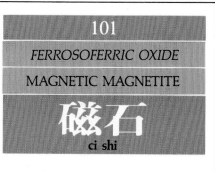

101
FERROSOFERRIC OXIDE
MAGNETIC MAGNETITE

磁石
ci shi

Natural distribution: Common mineral
Parts used: Crushed stone
Nature: Pungent; cold
Affinity: Liver, kidneys
Effects: Sedative; tonic to blood and kidneys
Indications: Hypertension; heart palpitations; insomnia; hysteria; traumatic shock; fright; asthma due to "empty" kidneys; dizziness; ringing in ears and deafness
Dosage: 7-15 g
Remarks: An effective treatment for prolapse of the rectum; appropriate sedative for patients with weak blood and kidneys

102
FOSSILISED BONES OF DINOSAURS AND REPTILES

DRAGON BONES

龍骨
long gu

Natural distribution: World-wide
Parts used: Crushed fossilised bones
Nature: Sweet and sour; neutral
Affinity: Heart, liver, kidneys
Effects: Sedative; calms excess liver-yang; astringent
Indications: Hypertension; insomnia; shock; fright; hysteria; dizziness; spermatorrhoea; leukorrhoea; diarrhoea
Dosage: 10-20 g
Remarks: Effective external styptic action on abscesses and other persistent sores

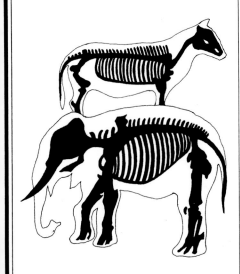

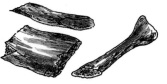

103
OSTREA RIVULARIS
(Ostreidae)

OYSTER SHELLS

牡蠣
mu li

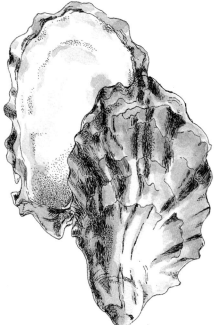

Natural distribution: World-wide
Parts used: Crushed or powdered shells
Nature: Salty and sour; slightly cold
Affinity: Liver, gall-bladder, kidneys
Effects: Sedative; calms excess liver-yang; astringent; softens and dissolves hard tumours
Indications: Hypertension; heart palpitations; insomnia; ascending excess liver-yang: dizziness, headache, blurry vision, etc.; severe fright; spasms; spermatorrhoea; menorrhagia; leukorrhoea; diarrhoea; cold-sweats; swollen lymph glands; hard tumours; vomiting bile
Dosage: 5-10 g
Remarks: Contains 75 percent calcium carbonate; promotes bone growth; prescribed for calcium-deficiency in pregnant women

104
ZIZIPHUS JUJUBA
(Rhamnaceae)

CHINESE JUJUBE

酸棗仁
suan zao ren

Natural distribution: China, Japan, India, Afghanistan, Malaysia
Parts used: Seeds
Nature: Sweet and sour; neutral
Affinity: Heart, spleen, liver, gall-bladder
Effects: Sedative to liver; cardiotonic; nutrient; tonic to yin; inhibits perspiration
Indications: Insomnia; neurasthenia; heart palpitations; cold sweats
Dosage: 6-15 g
Remarks: Long-term use improves the complexion

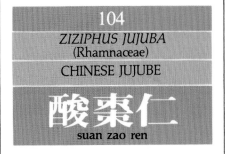

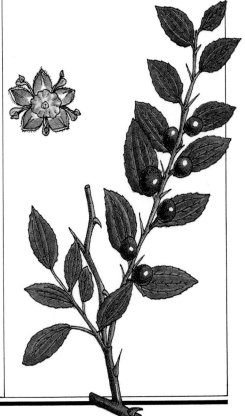

105
POLYGALA TENUIFOLIA
(Polygalaceae)

遠志
yuan zhi

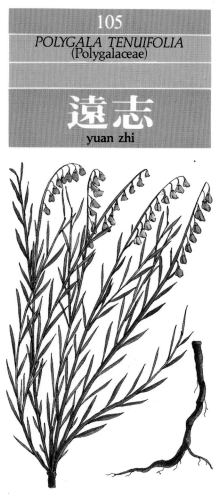

Natural distribution: Northern China, Mongolia
Parts used: Skin of the roots
Nature: Bitter and pungent; warm
Affinity: Lungs, heart, kidneys
Effects: Sedative; expectorant; tonic to heart and kidneys
Indications: Dizziness or fainting due to excess phlegm accumulation; insomnia; coughs with profuse phlegm
Dosage: 5-7 g
Remarks: The drug irritates the mucous membranes in the throat, causing hypersecretion and expectoration; combined with Chinese licorice, it is a good expectorant for heavy smokers

106
TRITICUM AESTIVUM
(Gramineae)
COMMON WHEAT

小麥
xiao mai

Natural distribution: Northern hemisphere
Parts used: Mature kernels
Nature: Sweet; neutral
Affinity: Heart
Effects: Sedative; cardiotonic;

Indications: Insomnia; hypertension
Dosage: 15-30 g
Remarks: The immature grain is prescribed to inhibit profuse sweating due to "empty" ailments

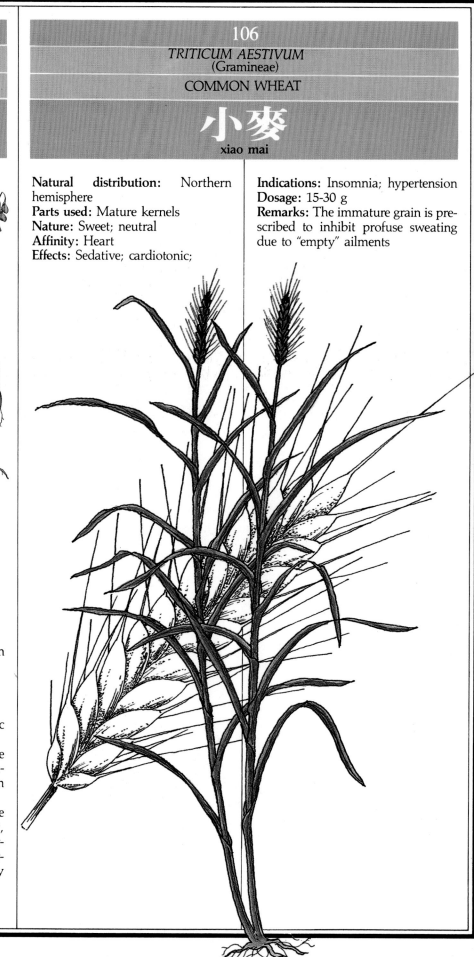

Liver Sedatives Or "Calm The Liver, Stop The Wind"

These drugs have specific affinity for the liver and function to "calm ascending liver-yang" and all its attendant nervous symptoms. Many serious nervous ailments are directly related to liver dysfunction. "Stop the wind" means to impede the nervous energy "wind" which emanates from a diseased or inflamed liver and injures other parts. Common symptoms of uncontrolled ascending "liver-wind" are blurry vision, nervous excitability, quick temper, convulsions, dizziness and delirium and other disorders of the central nervous system. Nervous disorders are often best remedied by highly toxic drugs.

These drugs must be carefully selected according to differential diagnosis to insure that the right type of liver sedative is chosen to match the specific causes of the liver's dysfunction. Patients with weak spleens and chronic spasmic conditions should avoid the cool and cold liver sedatives. Those with blood deficiency and yin-injuries should use the warm and hot liver sedatives sparingly.

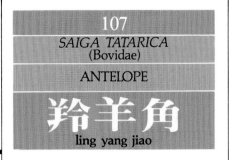

107
SAIGA TATARICA
(Bovidae)

ANTELOPE

羚羊角

ling yang jiao

Natural distribution: Northwestern China
Parts used: Horn
Nature: Salty; cold
Affinity: Liver
Effects: Sedative to liver; antipyretic; antispasmodic; improves vision
Indications: Symptoms of ascending liver-yang excess: giddyness, blurry vision, headache; convulsions and spasms; epilepsy; excess body heat; delirium; swollen, painful eyes
Dosage: 1.5-3 g
Remarks: The drug is very expensive today, so is generally prescribed as part of pill prescriptions, not brews; lowers blood pressure; effective preventive in strokes

108
HALIOTIS GIGANTEA
(Haliotidae)

SEA-EAR SHELLS

石决明

shi jue ming

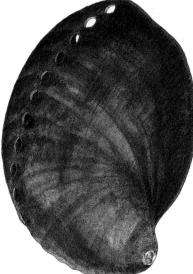

Natural distribution: World-wide
Parts used: Crushed or powdered shell
Nature: Salty, slightly cold
Affinity: Liver
Effects: Sedative to liver; antipyretic; improves vision
Indications: Dizziness, giddyness, blurry vision, painful and swollen eyes and other liver-yang ascending symptoms
Dosage: 15-30 g
Remarks: Especially effective remedy for cataracts

109 *GASTRODIA ELATA* (Orchidaceae)	110 *UNCARIA RHYNCHOPHYLLA* (Rubiaceae) MORNING STAR	111 *HEMATITE* BROWN IRON OXIDE
天麻 tian ma	鈎藤 gou teng	代赭石 dai zhe shi

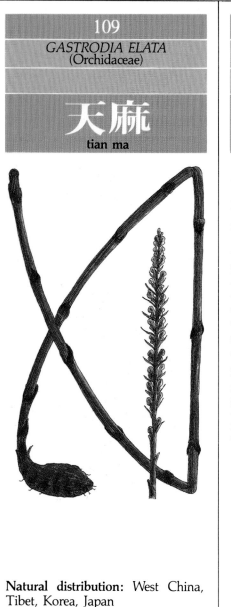

Uncaria Rhynchophylla (110)

Natural distribution: Central China
Parts used: Stem and spines
Nature: Sweet; slightly cold
Affinity: Liver, pericardium
Effects: Sedative to liver; antipyretic; antispasmodic in children's nervous disorders
Indications: Ailments of liver-yang ascending: pressure and pain in head, dizziness, blurry vision; body heat due to heat excess; convulsions and spasms in children; fainting and convulsions during the sixth, seventh and eighth month of pregnancy
Dosage: 5-10 g
Remarks: The drug dilates the capillaries and other blood vessels and is now used to lower blood pressure as well

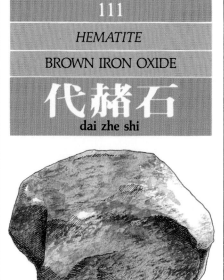

Hematite (111)

Natural distribution: Common mineral
Nature: Bitter; cold
Affinity: Liver, pericardium
Effects: Sedative to liver; antiemetic; hemostatic; tonic to blood; astringent
Indications: Hiccups, burps, nausea and vomiting; nosebleeds; ringing in ear, dizziness headaches due to ascending liver-yang
Dosage: 10-105 g
Remarks: The drug has also been found effective in bronchial asthma

Gastrodia Elata (109)

Natural distribution: West China, Tibet, Korea, Japan
Parts used: Rhizomes
Nature: Sweet; slightly warm
Affinity: Liver
Effects: Sedative to liver; clear the meridians
Indications: Giddyness and fainting due to liver inflammations; convulsions due to heat excess; headaches; numbness
Dosage: 5-10 g
Remarks: This drug is most effective against dizziness and giddyness due to liver inflammations

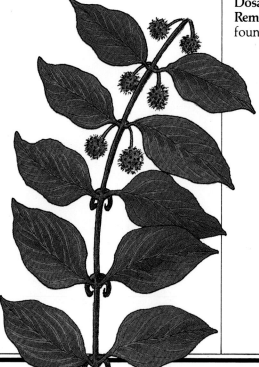

112	113	114
PHERETIMA ASPERGILLUM (Megascolecidae)	*BUTHUS MARTENSI* (Buthidae)	*SCOLOPENDRA SUBSPINIPES* (Scolopendridae)
COMMON EARTHWORM	SCORPION	CENTIPEDE
蚯蚓 qiu yin	蝎 xie	蜈蚣 wu gong

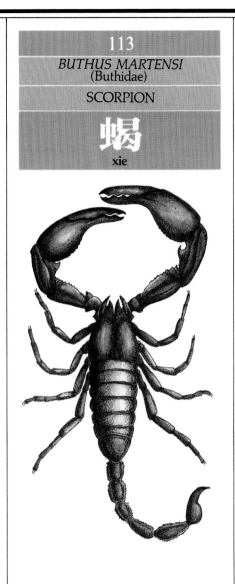

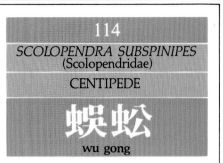

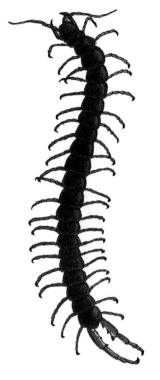

Natural distribution: World-wide
Nature: Salty; cold
Affinity: Stomach, spleen, liver, kidneys
Effects: Sedative to liver; antipyretic; clears the meridians; dilates bronchii; diuretic
Indications: Nervous convulsions; pains of "wind-damp;" stroke paralysis; asthma; difficult urination; swelling
Dosage: 5-10 g
Remarks: Lowers blood pressure; relaxes and softens hard arteries and veins

Natural distribution: World-wide
Parts used: Whole insect
Nature: Pungent; neutral
Affinity: Liver
Effects: Sedative to liver; tonic to nerves; antispasmodic; analgesic; antidote
Indications: Spasms and nervous convulsions; tetanus infection; headache and other pains of "wind-damp;" abscesses and boils
Dosage: Pure powder—0.05-0.1 g; brewed—1.5-3 g
Remarks: Poisonous

Natural distribution: World-wide
Parts used: Whole insect
Nature: Pungent; warm
Affinity: Liver
Effects: Sedative to liver; antispasmodic; antidote
Indications: Traumatic shock; fright; tetanus infection; externally applied to pus-abscesses and serious infections
Dosage: Pure powder—0.3-1 g; brewed—1-3 g
Remarks: Poisonous; antidote in poisonous snake-bites; ingredient in cancer prescriptions; should be avoided by pregnant women; antidote for centipede bites is juice of fresh mulberry leaves with salt applied directly to wound

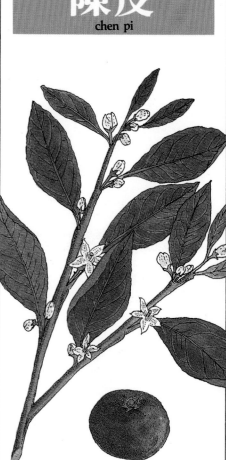

115
CITRUS RETICULATA
(Rutaceae)

MANDARIN ORANGE

陳皮
chen pi

ENERGY REGULATORS OR "MANAGE AND DISCIPLINE *QI*"

Drugs which regulate and balance the flow of vital-energies in the body and remedy illnesses due to energy imbalances are called "energy regulators." Such ailments are of two types: energy deficient and energy stagnant. Energy deficient ailments are treated with tonic medications, which appear under the "tonic" section. Energy stagnant ailments are treated with drugs which "manage and discipline *qi*."

Energy stagnation occurs when *qi* does not flow freely through the body's meridian network. *Qi* is literally "blocked" in the meridians, depriving the rest of the body of vital energy. Energy stagnation is caused by extreme imbalances between "hot" and "cold" energies, sudden emotional outbursts, poor diet, overeating, prolonged hunger, excess phlegm, damp excess, bruises and clots due to traumatic injuries.

Common symptoms of energy stagnation fall into three categories. Spleen and stomach energy stagnation: abdominal swelling and discomfort, poor appetite; dyspepsia, rising bile, nausea and vomiting, stomach aches, irregular bowel movements. Liver energy stagnation: pain and pressure in rib-cage, painful testicles and scrotum, dysmenorrhoea and swelling, pain, or tumours in breast. Lung energy stagnation: shortness of breath, irregular respiration, oppression in chest, cough, asthma.

Depending on the type of stagnation, these drugs have a variety of effects: they clear meridian blockages, alleviate pain, eliminate mental depression, facilitate energy flow, expand the chest cavity, scatter stagnant *qi*, suppress "rebellious *qi*," tonify the stomach, promote digestion and others.

The drugs are mostly "pungent" and "warm," properties which tend to scatter *qi*. Patients with energy- and yin-deficiencies should use them sparingly.

Natural distribution: Southeastern China, Taiwan, Vietnam
Parts used: Rind of the fruit
Nature: Pungent and bitter; warm
Affinity: Spleen, lungs
Effects: Regulates energy; digestive; stomachic; expectorant; antitussive; antiemetic; drying
Indications: Energy stagnation in spleen and stomach: abdominal pain and pressure, nausea and vomiting, dyspepsia, etc.; oppression in chest, cough, stagnation due to excess phlegm
Dosage: 3-8 g
Remarks: The rind contains Vitamins A, B, and C; the white fibres of the rind are the most effective parts as expectorants; the seeds are analgesic

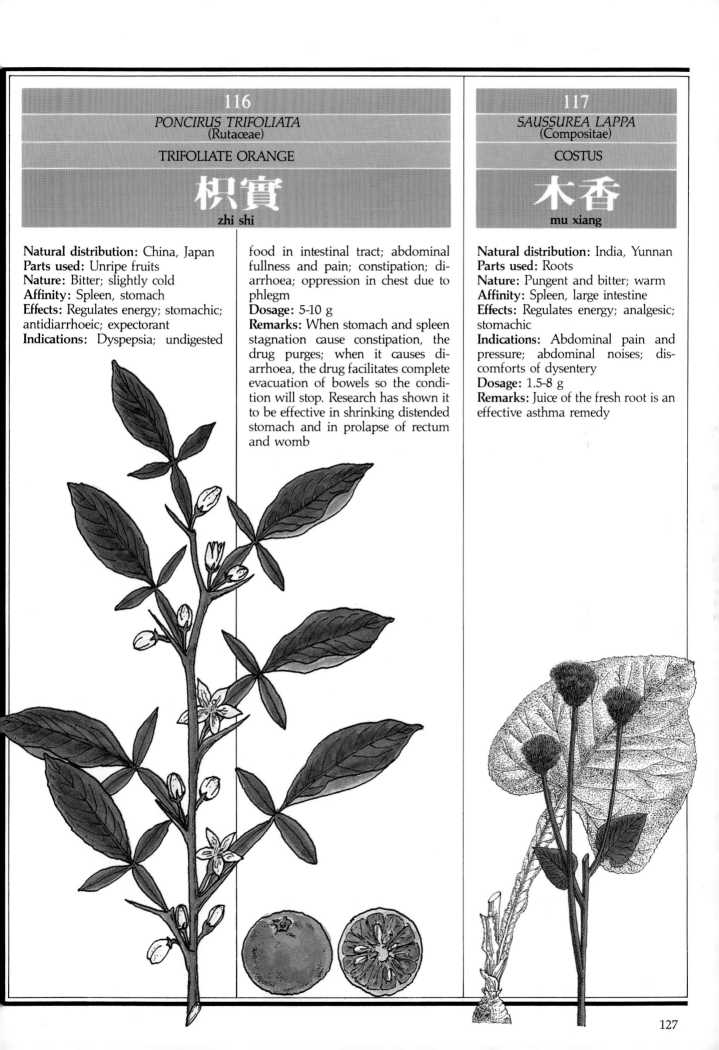

116

PONCIRUS TRIFOLIATA
(Rutaceae)

TRIFOLIATE ORANGE

枳實
zhi shi

Natural distribution: China, Japan
Parts used: Unripe fruits
Nature: Bitter; slightly cold
Affinity: Spleen, stomach
Effects: Regulates energy; stomachic; antidiarrhoeic; expectorant
Indications: Dyspepsia; undigested food in intestinal tract; abdominal fullness and pain; constipation; diarrhoea; oppression in chest due to phlegm
Dosage: 5-10 g
Remarks: When stomach and spleen stagnation cause constipation, the drug purges; when it causes diarrhoea, the drug facilitates complete evacuation of bowels so the condition will stop. Research has shown it to be effective in shrinking distended stomach and in prolapse of rectum and womb

117

SAUSSUREA LAPPA
(Compositae)

COSTUS

木香
mu xiang

Natural distribution: India, Yunnan
Parts used: Roots
Nature: Pungent and bitter; warm
Affinity: Spleen, large intestine
Effects: Regulates energy; analgesic; stomachic
Indications: Abdominal pain and pressure; abdominal noises; discomforts of dysentery
Dosage: 1.5-8 g
Remarks: Juice of the fresh root is an effective asthma remedy

118

CYPERUS ROTUNDUS
(Cyperaceae)

NUT GRASS

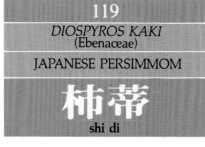

香附

xiang fu

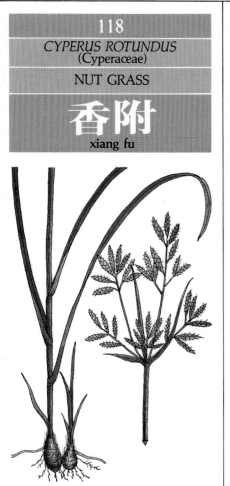

Natural distribution: Asia, Australia, America, Europe
Parts used: Roots and tubercles
Nature: Pungent, slightly bitter and sweet; neutral
Affinity: Liver, pericardium
Effects: Regulates liver energy; emmenagogue; sedative; analgesic
Indications: Liver energy stagnation: oppression in chest and pain in rib-cage, stomach ache, dyspepsia; amenorrhoea; dysmenorrhoea
Dosage: 5-10 g

119

DIOSPYROS KAKI
(Ebenaceae)

JAPANESE PERSIMMOM

柿蒂

shi di

Natural distribution: China, Japan, Vietnam, eastern India
Parts used: Peduncle
Nature: Bitter; neutral
Affinity: Stomach
Effects: Regulates stomach and spleen energy; controls hiccups and coughs
Indications: Hiccups
Dosage: 4-6 g
Remarks: For effective control of hiccups, use with clove and fresh ginger; the ripe, dried fruit is stomachic and astringent; the juice of the fresh, unripe fruits lowers blood pressure and is used in hypertension

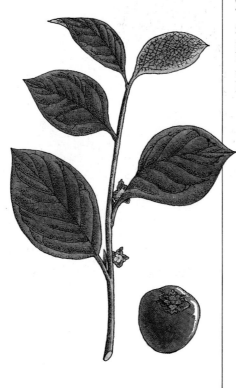

BLOOD REGULATORS OR "MANAGE AND DISCIPLINE BLOOD"

Drugs which facilitate blood circulation, dissolve clots and keep the blood vessels soft and supple are called "blood regulators." This category also includes hemostatic herbs which stop or prevent internal and external hemorrhage. They are used in ailments due to poor circulation—"blood stagnation"—blockages in the circulatory system, or uncontrolled hemorrhage.

Clot-dissolving and circulation-promoting drugs should only be used when the symptoms indicate stagnation or blockage in the bloodstream. The opposite acting hemostatic herbs are used in cases of hemorrhage, seepage, or other "leaks" in the circulatory system. The same drug, however, can have both effects, depending upon the dosage. These drugs have a strong affinity for the heart and/or liver, which are the two vital organs controlling blood. They are among the most useful and effective of all Chinese herbs.

120	121	122
SALVIA MILTIORRHIZA (Labiatae)	*LIGUSTICUM WALLICHII* (Umbelliferae)	*PRUNUS PERSICA* (Rosaceae)
		PEACH

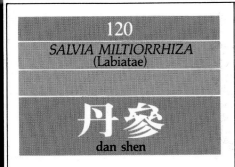

丹参
dan shen

川芎
chuan xiong

桃仁
tao ren

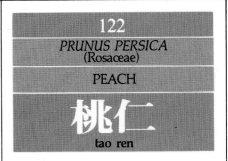

Natural distribution: Northeastern China, Manchuria, Japan
Parts used: Roots
Nature: Bitter; slightly cold
Affinity: Heart, pericardium
Effects: Promotes circulation; dissolves clots; refrigerant to blood; tonic to blood; sedative
Indications: Amenorrhoea; metrorrhagia; mastitis; post-natal abdominal pains; bodily pains due to poor circulation; acute pains in chest and abdomen; blood clots; heart palpitation; insomnia
Dosage: 5-6 g
Remarks: The drug is most commonly used in blood-related disorders in women; it is also antiphlogistic to the liver; excellent for coronary diseases

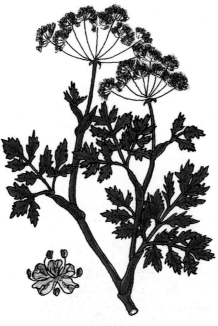

Natural distribution: China, Europe, North America
Parts used: Kernel of the pits
Nature: Bitter and sweet; neutral
Affinity: Heart, liver, large intestine
Effects: Promotes circulation; dissolves clots; laxative; emollient; antitussive
Indications: Amenorrhoea; dysmenorrhoea; post-natal abdominal pain; accumulated blood clots; blood seepage; traumatic injuries; pain and pressure in rib-cage; constipation due to dry intestines
Dosage: 5-10 g
Remarks: Also effective against high blood pressure and chronic appendicitis; high doses are toxic

Natural distribution: Sichuan, Yunnan, Guangdong
Parts used: Roots
Nature: Pungent; warm
Affinity: Liver, gall-bladder, pericardium
Effects: Promotes circulation; regulates energy; emmenagogue; analgesic; sedative
Indications: Amenorrhoea; dysmenorrhoea; post-natal abdominal pain; traumatic injury; painful abscesses; "wind-damp" discomfort; headaches due to colds
Dosage: 4-11 g
Remarks: The drug dilates the capillaries and other blood vessels and thus lowers blood pressure

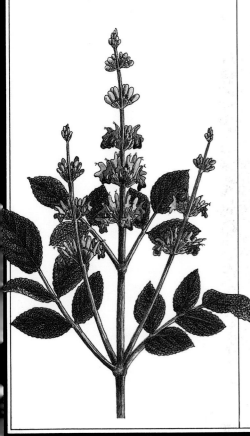

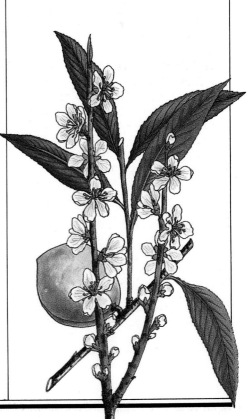

123	124	125
CARTHAMUS TINCTORIUS (Compositae)	*ACHYRANTHES BIDENTATA* (Amarantaceae)	*MANIS PENTADACTYLA* (Manidae)
SAFFLOWER		PANGOLIN

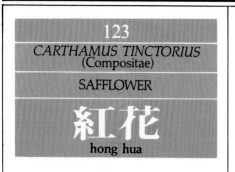

紅花

hong hua

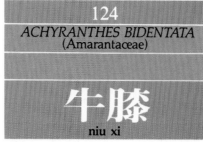

牛膝

niu xi

穿山甲

chuan shan jia

Natural distribution: China, Indochina, Tibet
Parts used: Flowers
Nature: Pungent; warm
Affinity: Heart, liver
Effects: Promotes circulation; dissolves clots; emennagogue; astringent
Indications: Amenorrhoea; dysmenorrhoea, post-natal abdominal pain; clots or seepages of blood in abdominal region; traumatic injuries; stiffness and pain in joints
Dosage: 2-5 g
Remarks: The extracted oil of the herb is used in *tui na* massage; pregnant women should avoid the drug

Natural distribution: China, Indochina, India, Sri Lanka, Malaysia, Indonesia
Parts used: Roots
Nature: Bitter and sour; neutral
Affinity: Liver, kidneys
Effects: Promotes circulation; dissolves clots; emmenagogue; tonic to liver and kidneys; nourishes sinews and bones; diuretic
Indications: Amenorrhoea; dysmenorrhoea; traumatic injuries; stiffness and pain in lower back and loins; weak legs and feet; blood in vomit, sputum and nosebleeds; painful or bleeding gums; urethritis
Dosage: 5-10 g

Natural distribution: Southern China, Vietnam, Taiwan
Parts used: Scales
Nature: Salty; slightly cold
Affinity: Liver, stomach
Effects: Promotes circulation; emmenagogue; promotes lactation and secretion; reduces swelling; dispels pus
Indications: Amenorrhoea; insufficient lactation; discomforts of "wind-damp"; tight, painful joints and sinews; promotes suppuration in skin ailments
Dosage: 5-10 g
Remarks: This drug promotes growth of white blood cells, which have been shown to produce the potent curative agent interferon

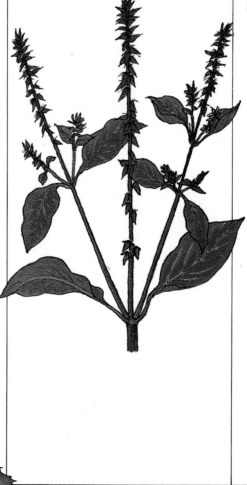

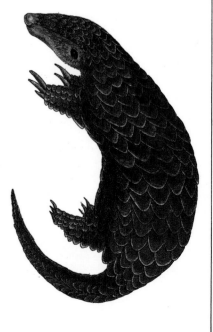

126	127	128
BOSWELLIA CARTERII (Burseraceae)	*CURCUMA AROMATICA* (Zingiberaceae)	*AGRIMONIA PILOSA* (Rosaceae)
MASTIC TREE	WILD TURMERIC	AGRIMONY

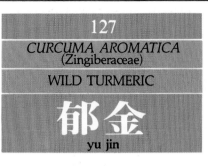

乳香

ru xiang

郁金

yu jin

龍芽草

long ya cao

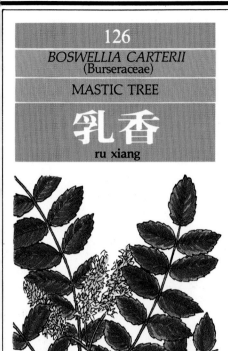

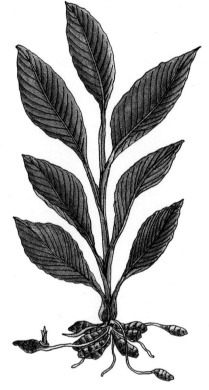

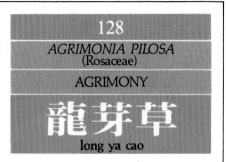

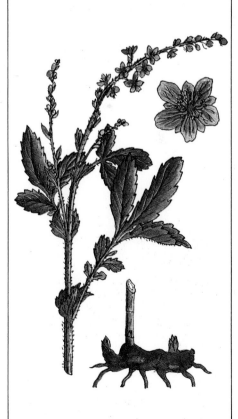

Natural distribution: China, Japan, Korea, Taiwan, Europe
Parts used: Leaves and stems
Nature: Bitter; cool
Affinity: Lungs, liver, spleen
Effects: Astringent; hemostatic
Indications: All forms of hemorrhage
Dosage: 10-30 g
Remarks: The drug increases the number of thrombocytes (blood-clotting cells), which improves coagulation capacity by 40-50 percent; it strengthens osmotic resistance of blood vessel walls; it is cardiotonic

Natural distribution: Mediterranean area
Parts used: Solid, resinous exudation beneath the bark
Nature: Pungent and bitter; warm
Affinity: Heart, liver, spleen
Effects: Promotes circulation; analgesic; antitussive; promotes growth of muscle
Indications: Amenorrhoea; dysmenorrhoea; traumatic injury; lower abdominal pains; "wind-damp" discomforts; externally applied to stubborn abscesses, boils and carbuncles
Dosage: 3-6 g
Remarks: Used as gargle to eliminate bad breath

Natural distribution: India, Indochina, Taiwan
Parts used: Roots
Nature: Pungent and bitter; cold
Affinity: Heart, lungs, liver
Effects: Hemostatic; dissolves clots; refrigerant to blood; nourishes the gall-bladder; stimulant to gall-bladder
Indications: Pressure and pain in chest; semi-conscious states; traumatic shock; hysteria; acute, sharp pains in rib-cage; amenorrhoea; dysmenorrhoea; blood in vomit, urine and nosebleeds; jaundice
Dosage: 5-10 g
Remarks: This is one of the drugs which both stop hemorrhage and dissolve clots

129	130	131
BLETILLA STRIATA (Orchidaceae)	*ARTEMISIA VULGARIS* (Compositae)	*CIRSIUM JAPONICUM* (Compositae)
BLETILLA	MUGWORT	TIGER THISTLE

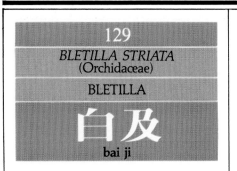

白及

bai ji

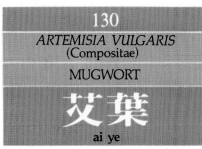

艾葉

ai ye

大薊

da ji

129 — BLETILLA

Natural distribution: China, Indochina
Parts used: Tubers
Nature: Bitter, sweet and sour; slightly cold
Affinity: Liver, lungs, stomach
Effects: Astringent; hemostatic; reduces swelling; promotes healing of flesh
Indications: Blood in vomit, sputum and nosebleeds; external application to traumatic injuries, skin infections and abscesses
Dosage: Pure powder—1-3 g;
brewed—3-8 g
Remarks: For external use, the drug is powdered and mixed with sesame oil; it is astringent and emollient to burns, abscesses and other skin irritations; it is highly hemostatic in bleeding wounds; internally, it is most effective in stomach and lung hemorrhages

130 — MUGWORT

Natural distribution: China, Asia, Europe
Parts used: Leaves
Nature: Bitter and pungent; warm
Affinity: Liver, spleen, kidneys
Effects: Hemostatic; astringent; warms the meridians; analgesic; dispels internal cold
Indications: Blood in vomit, sputum and stool; nosebleeds; menorrhagia (vaginal bleeding): excess menses, bleeding during pregnancy; dysmenorrhoea
Dosage: 5-10 g
Remarks: This herb is the main source of moxa used in moxibustion

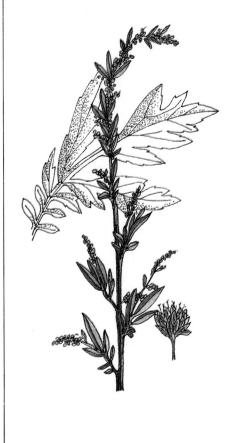

131 — TIGER THISTLE

Natural distribution: China, Japan, Vietnam
Parts used: Whole plant
Nature: Sweet; cold
Affinity: Liver
Effects: Hemostatic; refrigerant to blood
Indications: Blood in sputum, vomit, urine and nosebleeeds; menorrhagia
Dosage: 10-15 g
Remarks: Effective remedy for high blood pressure; externally, the pulverised leaves are applied to scaly skin diseases

132	133	134
THUJA ORIENTALIS (Cupressaceae)	*SOPHORA JAPONICA* (Leguminosae)	*SANGUISORBA OFFICINALIS* (Rosaceae)
ARBOR-VITAE	PAGODA TREE	GARDEN BURNET

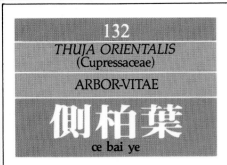

側柏葉
ce bai ye

槐花
huai hua

地楡
di yu

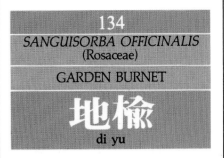

132 — ARBOR-VITAE

Natural distribution: China, Japan, India

Parts used: Leaves and stems

Nature: Bitter and sour; slightly cold

Affinity: Lungs, liver, large intestine

Effects: Hemostatic; astringent; refrigerant to blood; emmenagogue; antipyretic

Indications: All forms of hemorrhage

Dosage: 5-10 g

Remarks: The seeds are used as sedative in insomnia, heart palpitation and nervous disorders; the fresh leaves steeped for 7 days in 60 percent alcohol solution produce a potion which is rubbed on bald spots 3 times a day to promote hair growth

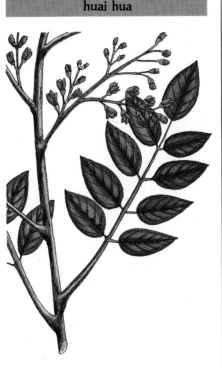

134 — GARDEN BURNET

Natural distribution: China, northern Asia, northern Europe

Parts used: Roots

Nature: Bitter and sour; slightly cold

Affinity: Liver, large intestine

Effects: Hemostatic; astringent; refrigerant to blood

Indications: Blood in stool and urine; bleeding dysentery; bleeding hemmorrhoids; menorrhagia

Dosage: 3-10 g

Remarks: The fresh root is pulverised, mixed with sesame oil and applied to burns, pruritus and eczema

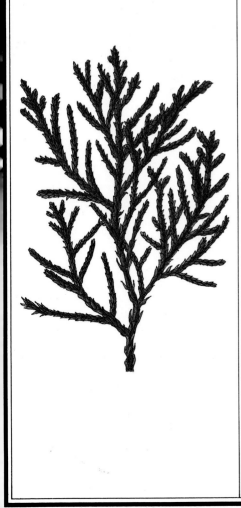

133 — PAGODA TREE

Natural distribution: China, Korea, Vietnam

Parts used: Flowers or flower buds

Nature: Bitter, slightly cold

Affinity: Liver, large intestine

Effects: Hemostatic; refrigerant to blood; dissolves clots and cholesterol

Indications: Blood in stool; bleeding dysentery; bleeding hemmorrhoids; menorrhagia; blood in vomit, sputum and nosebleeds

Dosage: 9-15 g

Remarks: Recent new uses for the flowers are to lower blood pressure and as preventive in cerebral hemorrhage (10-15 g infusion per day); the drug strengthens and tonifies the walls of capillaries to prevent seepage; the seeds are effective against bleeding hemmorrhoids and bloody stool

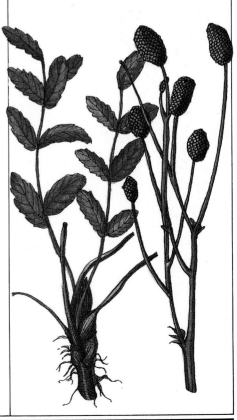

135

RUBIA CORDIFOLIA
(Rubiaceae)

INDIAN MADDER

茜草根
qian cao gen

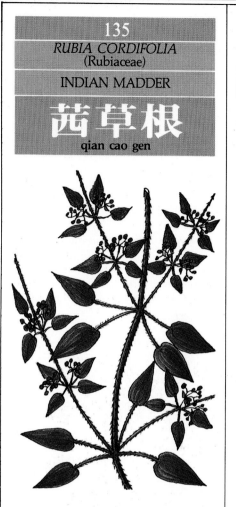

Natural distribution: China, India, Africa

Parts used: Roots

Nature: Bitter; cold

Affinity: Liver

Effects: Hemostatic; refrigerant to blood; dissolves clots and cholesterol; emmenagogue

Indications: All types of hemorrhage; amenorrhoea; post-natal bleeding; traumatic injuries

Dosage: 5-10 g

Remarks: The drug has hemostatic properties in small doses (5-10 g) and clot-dissolving properties in high doses (over 20 g); its hemostatic action is greatly enhanced if the herb is first dry-fried in a hot pan with lumps of charcoal

136

TYPHA LATIFOLIA
(Typhaceae)

COMMON CATTAIL

香蒲
xiang pu

Natural distribution: Northern China, northern Europe, North America

Parts used: Pollen

Nature: Sweet; neutral

Affinity: Liver, pericardium

Effects: Hemostatic; astringent; promotes circulation and dissolves clots; diuretic

Indications: Blood in vomit, urine and stools; coughing blood; nosebleeds; menorrhagia; traumatic injuries; pain and pressure in heart region; post-natal abdominal pain; dysmenorrhoea

Dosage: 4-8 g

Remarks: The plain herb promotes circulation and dissolves clots; dry-fried with lumps of charcoal, it becomes highly hemostatic

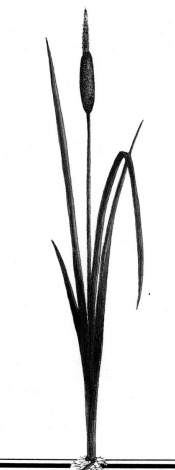

137

PANAX NOTOGINSENG
(Araliaceae)

NOTOGINSENG

三七
san qi

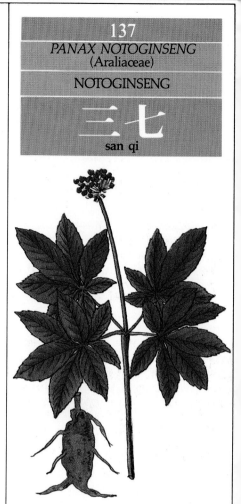

Natural distribution: Yunnan, Sichuan, Japan

Parts used: Roots

Nature: Sweet and slightly bitter; warm

Affinity: Liver, stomach

Effects: Hemostatic; promotes circulation; dissolves clots; analgesic

Indications: Coughing blood; blood in stool; nosebleeds; traumatic injuries

Dosage: Pure powder—1-2 g; brewed—5-10 g

Remarks: Extremely effective styptic action when applied directly to traumatic wounds; heals without leaving clots and scars; internally and externally, best drug for serious bleeding; can be used safely in large doses

STOMACHIC, DIGESTIVE OR "DIGEST AND GUIDE"

Stomachics and digestives are those herbs which tonify the stomach and spleen, promote digestion, facilitate distribution, and accelerate movement of accumulated excess food in the stomach. Digestive ailments requiring treatment with these medications are indicated by symptoms of oppression and swelling in abdomen, belching, coughing up bile, nausea and vomiting, irregular bowel movements, dyspepsia, and all "empty" spleen and stomach symptoms. In cases of "empty" spleen and stomach, stomachic herbs should be combined with spleen tonics. In cases of "cold" in spleen and stomach, use with drugs which are "warming" to interior. When the digestive problems are due to damp-excess, combine with aromatic "moisture transforming" herbs. When energy stagnation is the source of problems, use in combination with energy regulating herbs. If symptoms include constipation, include cathartics in the treatment.

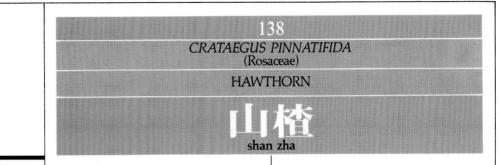

138
CRATAEGUS PINNATIFIDA
(Rosaceae)

HAWTHORN

山楂
shan zha

Natural distribution: Eastern China, Japan
Parts used: Fruits
Nature: Sweet and sour; slightly warm
Affinity: Spleen, stomach, liver
Effects: Digestive; stomachic; moves stagnant excess food; antidiarrhoeic
Indications: Stagnant, undigested food accumulated in stomach; excess consumption of meats and fats; diarrhoea; post-natal abdominal pain; scrotal pain and pressure
Dosage: 6-15 g
Remarks: The drug is especially effective in promoting digestion and movement of meats and fats; it dilates the blood vessels to lower blood pressure; dissolves cholesterol deposits in lining of blood vessels

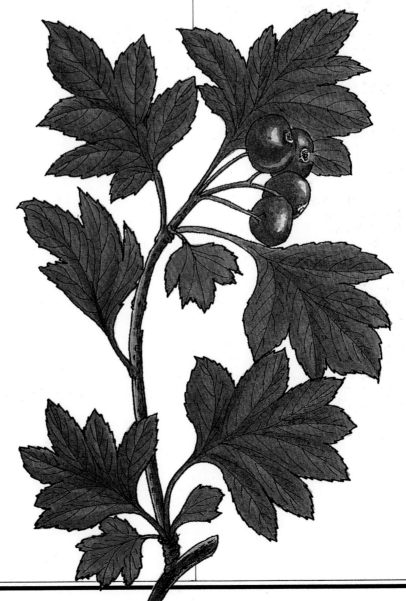

GALLUS GALLUS DOMESTICUS
(Phasianidae)

CHICKEN

雞內金

ji nei jin

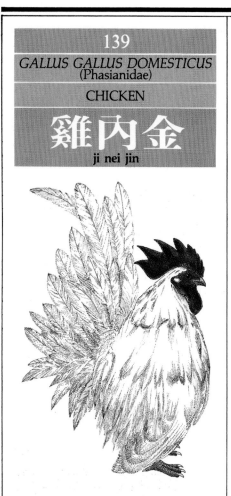

Natural distribution: Common world-wide

Parts used: Gastric tissue from gizzard

Nature: Sweet; neutral

Affinity: Spleen, stomach, small intestine, bladder

Effects: Stomachic; digestive; moves accumulated excess food in stomach

Indications: Stagnant, undigested food in stomach; oppressive, full feeling in abdomen; gastroenteritis; urinal incontinence; spermatorrhoea

Dosage: 4-8 g

Remarks: Dry-fried with lumps of charcoal and powdered, it is applied to painful abscesses in the mouth

---

HORDEUM VULGARE
(Gramineae)

BARLEY

麥芽

mai ya

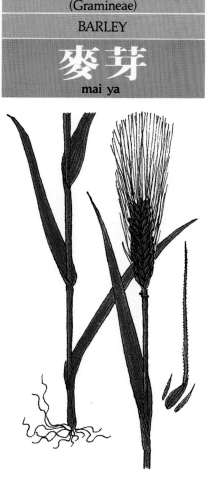

Natural distribution: China, Europe, America

Parts used: Dried, germinated sprouts

Nature: Salty; neutral

Affinity: Spleen, stomach

Effects: Stomachic; digestive; suppresses lactation

Indications: Stagnant, undigested food in stomach; pressure and fullness in abdomen; loss of appetite due to weak spleen and stomach; excess lactation; weaning

Dosage: 10-20 g

Remarks: The herb has abortifacient properties which facilitate contractions during childbirth; it is especially effective in promoting digestion and movement of grains and vegetables

---

EXPECTORANTS AND ANTITUSSIVES OR "MELT MUCUS, STOP COUGHS"

Medicines which facilitate the bringing up or the transformation of phlegm from the respiratory tract are called "expectorant." Those which control coughing and soothe the throat are called "antitussive." Expectorants generally have antitussive action and vice versa, which is why they appear under the same heading. Expectorants are used not only against excess phlegm due to coughs and colds, but also against other phlegm excess related ailments such as goitre, swelling of the lymph glands, epilepsy, certain types of fainting spells and others.

In clinical applications of these herbs, attention should be paid to the following points: both internal and external ailments can induce excess phlegm accumulation and coughing. When selecting expectorants and antitussives for therapeutic use, they must be combined with other types of herbs appropriate to the original causes of the problem. Phlegm and coughs due to external ailments should be treated in combination with diaphoretic herbs which "release externally"; "empty" ailments should be treated in combination with tonifying medications. When there is blood in the phlegm, avoid using expectorants of a highly drying nature, which would increase blood seepage. While coughing is one of the early symptoms of measles, do not use warm or astringent antitussives in such cases.

141
PINELLIA TERNATA
(Araceae)

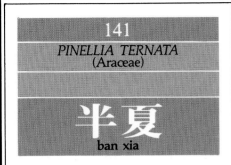

半夏

ban xia

Natural distribution: Southern China, Japan
Parts used: Tubers
Nature: Pungent; warm
Affinity: Spleen, stomach
Effects: Expectorant; antiemetic; drying; prevents hardening of spleen
Indications: Nausea and vomiting; chronic coughs; excess phlegm; gastritis
Dosage: 3-7 g
Remarks: Pregnant women should use herb sparingly; the fresh herb is slightly toxic, but the dried is not; the toxin is neutralised with tea or vinegar

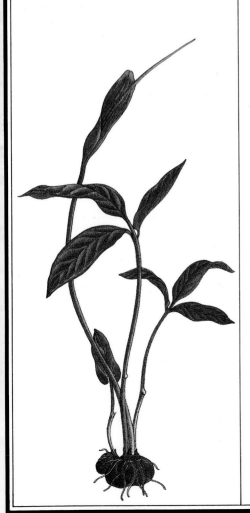

142
ARISAEMA CONSANGUINEUM
(Araceae)

天南星

tian nan xing

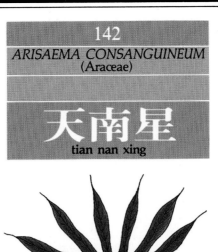

Natural distribution: Northern China, Korea, Japan
Parts used: Tubers
Nature: Pungent and bitter; warm
Affinity: Lungs, liver, spleen
Effects: Expectorant; drying; antispasmodic; analgesic
Indications: Coughs; heavy, lumpy phlegm; gastritis; dizziness and fainting due to excess phlegm; epilepsy; tetanus infections
Dosage: 3-10 g
Remarks: The fresh drug is toxic, but not the dried; when used fresh, it is mixed with beef bile or *Pinellia ternata* to neutralise its toxins

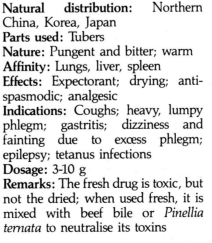

143
PERILLA FRUTESCENS
(Labiatae)

BEEFSTEAK PLANT

紫蘇子

zi su zi

Natural distribution: Southern China, Taiwan, Indochina, India
Parts used: Seeds
Nature: Pungent; warm
Affinity: Lungs
Effects: Antitussive; expectorant; asthma preventive; laxative
Indications: Excess phlegm; coughs; asthma; constipation due to dry intestines
Dosage: 5-8 g
Remarks: Leaves also used as diaphoretic and antitussive

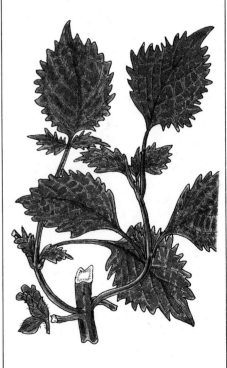

144	145	146
PLATYCODON GRANDIFLORUM (Campanulaceae)	*INULA BRITANNICA* (Compositae)	*CYNANCHUM STAUNTONI* (Asclepiadaceae)
BALLOON FLOWER	YELLOW STARWORT	DOG'S BANE
桔梗	旋覆花	白前
jie geng	xuan fu hua	bai qian

Natural distribution: China, Japan
Parts used: Roots
Nature: Bitter and pungent; neutral
Affinity: Lungs
Effects: Expectorant; dilates the bronchii; eliminates pus
Indications: Coughs; excess phlegm; sore throat; lung ulcers; throat ulcers
Dosage: 3-5 g
Remarks: The drug induces secretion of mucus in the throat to dilute accumulations of hard phlegm and facilitate bringing it up

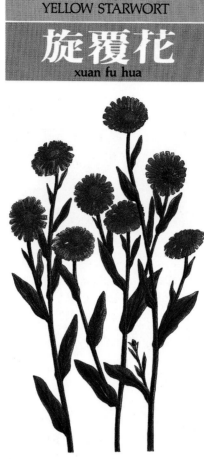

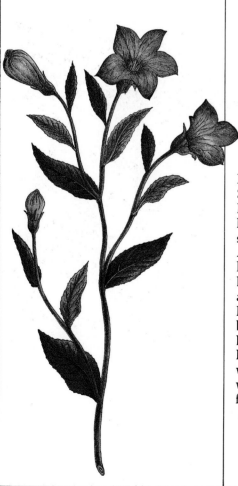

Natural distribution: China, Japan, Siberia, Europe
Parts used: Flowers
Nature: Bitter, pungent and salty; slightly warm
Affinity: Lungs, spleen, stomach, large intestine
Effects: Expectorant; antitussive; antiemetic
Indications: Coughs; excess phlegm, burping; nausea and vomiting
Dosage: 3-10 g
Remarks: This drug should be wrapped in a cheesecloth pouch when boiling to prevent irritating fibres from entering the broth

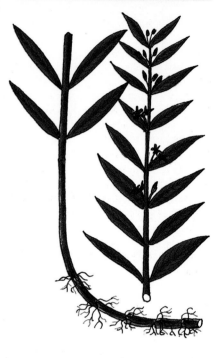

Natural distribution: Southern China,
Parts used: Pungent and sweet; slightly warm
Nature: Lungs
Affinity: Antitussive; expectorant; antiemetic
Effects: Coughs; excess phlegm; acute asthma
Indications: Dosage: 3-6 g

147	148	149
FRITILLARIA VERTICILLATA (Liliaceae)	*PEUCEDANUM DECURSIVUM* (Umbelliferae)	*TRICHOSANTHES KIRILOWII* (Cucurbitaceae) SNAKE GOURD

貝母
bei mu

前胡
qian hu

瓜蔞
gua lou

Natural distribution: Central China, Japan
Parts used: Corms
Nature: Bitter and sweet; slightly cold
Affinity: Heart, lungs
Effects: Antitussive; expectorant; antipyretic; scatters blockage and softens hard tissues
Indications: Chronic coughs; dry throat; "wind-heat" coughs; heavy, yellow phlegm; swelling of lymph glands; infected abscesses; lung and breast tumours
Dosage: Pure powder—1-2 g;
decoction—5-10 g
Remarks: The variety from Sichuan is superior

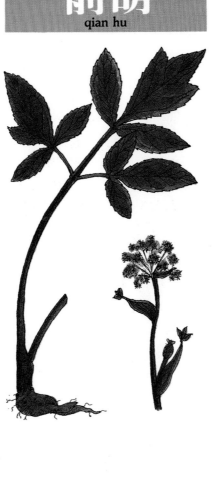

Natural distribution: Southern China, Vietnam
Parts used: Kernels of the seeds
Nature: Sweet; cold
Affinity: Lungs, stomach, large intestine
Effects: Expectorant; dilates bronchii; emollient; laxative
Indications: Coughs due to excess heat in lungs; heavy, yellow phlegm; lung tumours; pains in chest and rib-cage; breast tumours; constipation due to dry intestines
Dosage: 10-15 g
Remarks: The root is antipyretic, and it promotes lactation

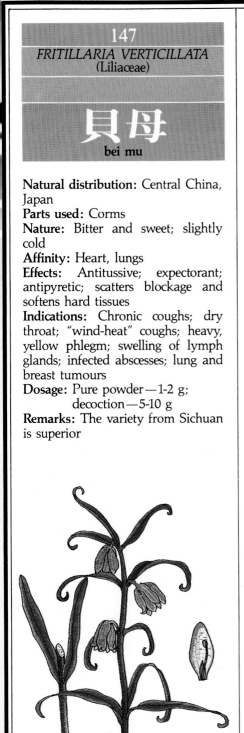

Natural distribution: Eastern China, Japan
Parts used: Roots
Nature: Bitter and pungent; slightly cold
Affinity: Lungs
Effects: Antitussive; expectorant; antiemetic; antipyretic; diaphoretic
Indications: Accumulations of excess heavy phlegm; coughs; asthma; bronchitis
Dosage: 3-10 g
Remarks: Induces secretion of mucus in respiratory tract to dilute hard phlegm in bronchial tubes and facilitate bringing it up

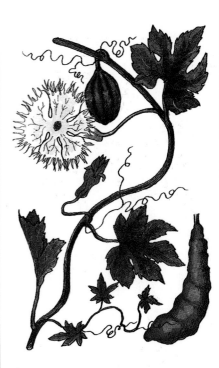

150	151	152
LEPIDIUM APETALUM (Cruciferae)	*SARGASSUM FUSIFORME* (Sargassaceae) GULF SEAWEED	*PRUNUS ARMENIACA* (Rosaceae) APRICOT
葶藶子 ting li zi	海藻 hai zao	杏仁 xing ren

151

Natural distribution: Coasts of China and Japan
Parts used: Whole plant
Nature: Bitter and salty; cold
Affinity: Liver, stomach, kidneys
Effects: Expectorant; diuretic; scatters goiter swellings
Indications: Swellings of lymph glands; goiter; excess hard lumpy phlegm
Dosage: 6-12 g
Remarks: The herb contains 0.2 percent iodine and has been used for centuries in ailments due to iodine deficiency

152

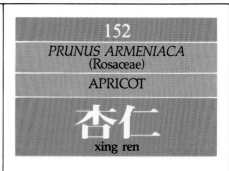

Natural distribution: Northwestern China
Parts used: Kernels of the pits
Nature: Sweet and bitter; warm
Affinity: Lungs, large intestine
Effects: Antitussive; sedative in asthma and bronchitis; laxative
Indications: Coughs; asthma; bronchitis; constipation due to dry intestines
Dosage: 4-10 g
Remarks: Mildly poisonous; toxic doses can be neutralised with a decoction of the rough outer bark of the tree

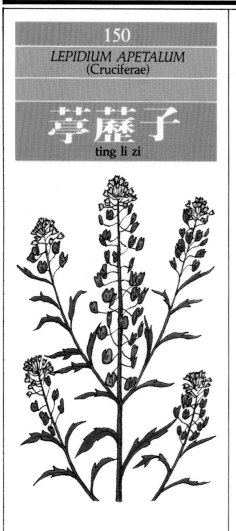

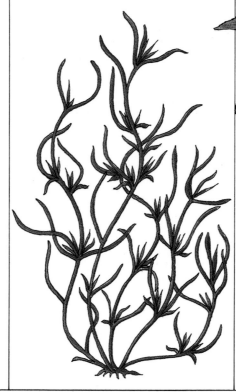

150

Natural distribution: Northwestern China, northern Asia, northern Europe, North America
Parts used: Seeds
Nature: Pungent and bitter; very cold
Affinity: Lungs, bladder
Effects: Expectorant; diuretic; reduces swelling; sedative in asthma and bronchitis
Indications: Excess phlegm; coughs; asthma; facial paralysis; water-retention in chest and abdomen
Dosage: 4-10 g

153	154	155
ARISTOLOCHIA DEBILIS (Aristolochiaceae)	*ERIOBOTRYA JAPONICA* (Rosaceae)	*TUSSILAGO FARFARA* (Compositae)
A CREEPING VINE	LOQUAT	COLTSFOOT

馬兜鈴
ma dou ling

枇杷葉
pi pa ye

款冬花
kuan dong hua

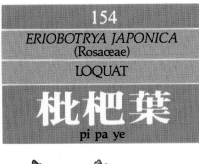

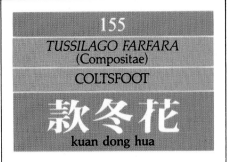

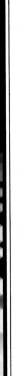

Natural distribution: Northern China, Europe, Africa
Parts used: Flowers and floral buds
Nature: Pungent; warm
Affinity: Lungs
Effects: Antitussive; expectorant
Indications: Coughs; asthma; chronic coughs due to "empty" lungs
Dosage: 3-10 g

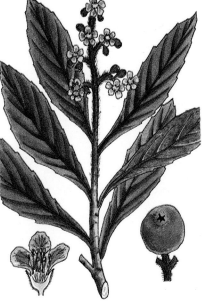

Natural distribution: Southwestern China, Japan, Indonesia; Europe
Parts used: Leaves
Nature: Bitter; neutral
Affinity: Lungs, stomach
Effects: Antitussive; expectorant; antiemetic
Indications: Coughs due to heat excess in lungs; difficult respiration; chronic burping; nausea and vomiting; thirst
Dosage: 10-15 g

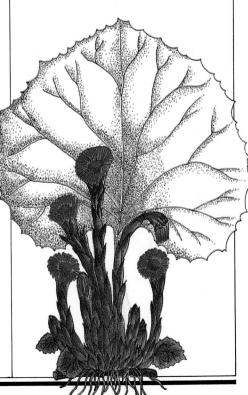

Natural distribution: Northern China, Japan
Parts used: Fruits
Nature: Bitter and slightly pungent; cold
Affinity: Lungs, large intestine
Effects: Antitussive; expectorant
Indications: Coughs due to excess heat in lungs; excess phlegm; irregular breathing; asthma; bronchitis; chronic coughs; blood in phlegm
Dosage: 3-10 g
Remarks: Mildly poisonous

141

156	157	158
ASTER TATARICUS (Compositae)	*STEMONA TUBEROSA* (Stemonaceae)	*DATURA METEL* (Solanaceae)
TARTARIAN ASTER		JIMSON WEED, LOCO WEED

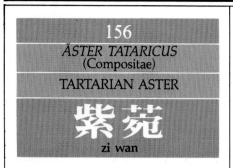

紫菀

zi wan

百部

bai bu

洋金花

yang jin hua

Natural distribution: Northern China, Siberia, Japan
Parts used: Roots
Nature: Pungent and bitter; warm
Affinity: Lungs
Effects: Antitussive; expectorant
Indications: Coughs, irregular breathing; accumulated excess phlegm; chronic coughs due to "empty" lungs
Dosage: 4-10 g
Remarks: The drug's primary effects are expectorant, not antitussive

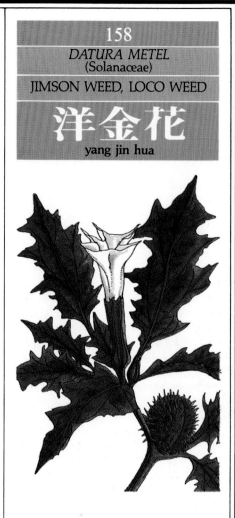

Natural distribution: Central China, Indochina, Taiwan, India
Parts used: Roots
Nature: Sweet and bitter; slightly cold
Affinity: Lungs
Effects: Antitussive; demulcent to lungs; anthelmintic; kills lice
Indications: Coughs; chronic, dry coughs; whooping cough; tapeworm; external application to lice
Dosage: 5-10 g
Remarks: Recent applications have found the drug to be effective against tuberculosis

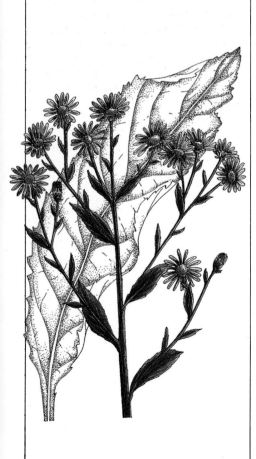

Natural distribution: Southern China, southern Asia, America
Parts used: Flowers
Nature: Pungent; warm
Affinity: Lung
Effects: Antitussive; sedative in asthma; analgesic
Indications: Asthma; irregular or difficult breathing; shortness of breath; stomach ache
Dosage: 0.1-0.25 g
Remarks: Poisonous; the dried flowers are smoked in a pipe to relieve asthma without phlegm excess; not suitable for use in children; traditionally, the drug has been used as a local anaesthetic before topical surgery; the leaves and seeds are used as local anaesthetics as well

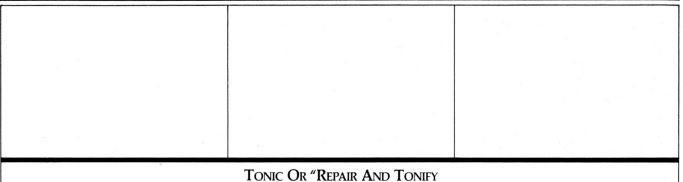

TONIC OR "REPAIR AND TONIFY EMPTINESS"

Herbs which restore strength and tonify weakened tissues when the body is "empty"—deficient—are called "tonic." They are used to repair damage caused by "empty" ailments. Clinically, tonics are used for two purposes. One is to increase the body's resistance to disease when resistance has been impaired by excess "evil-*qi*". Combined with drugs which dispel excess "evil-*qi*," tonics are used in ailments caused by excess "evil-*qi*" or deficient "pure-*qi*." They tend to restore the body's original primordial energies. The second clinical use is to restore energy and accelerate recovery in patients who have become weak and vulnerable due to long-standing chronic ailments. Tonics are among the most useful of all drugs in Chinese herbal medicine.

Tonics are primarily used in "empty" ailments, which are divided into four types: energy deficient, blood deficient, yang-deficient, and yin-deficient. Tonics are thus similarly sub-classified as energy tonics, blood nourishers, yang-tonics, and yin-nourishers. "Tonic" and "nourish" are interchangeable terms, though customarily "tonic" is used to describe yang and energy herbs, while "nourish" is used for yin and blood herbs.

In clinical application, it is important to match the right type of tonic to the equivalent type of deficiency, such as using yang-tonics for yang-deficiency, and so forth. Energy deficiency and yang deficiency are interrelated (energy belongs to yang) and their symptoms often appear together. Degeneration of vital energies and impairment of vital functions are the main indicators. Similarly, blood deficient and yin-deficient ailments often coincide (blood belongs to yin), and their main symptoms involve internal damage to the body's vital fluids and fluid balance. Therefore, energy- and yang-tonics are often combined in therapy, as are blood- and yin-nourishers. In cases of both blood and energy deficiency, or combined yin- and yang-deficiency, both types of tonics are applied.

In patients who have not fully recovered from "full" ailments, restorative tonics should be used sparingly in order to avoid retention of some of the "full-evil" excess.

Energy tonics or "tonify *qi*"

These tonics are used against ailments caused by energy *qi*-deficiency. They primarily tonify lung energy and spleen energy, where energy deficiencies usually come to rest. The spleen regulates digestion and distribution, and when it is

"empty," common symptoms are fatigue, loose and lumpy bowel movements, poor appetite, abdominal pain and pressure, hernias, prolapse of rectum, and others. The lungs regulate *qi*. When they are "empty", common symptoms are lack of energy, shallow and strained breathing, aversion to talk, slow and sluggish movements, cold sweats, and others. Energy tonics are used in all the above ailments and symptoms.

In therapy, energy tonics are often used together with blood nourishers because "*qi* is the general of the blood" and regulates its production and its circulation. Thus, when *qi* is deficient, blood also suffers. In cases of extreme blood deficiency, such as due to profuse loss of blood, energy tonics are used with blood nourishers to facilitate renewed blood production.

Excess or prolonged use of energy tonics may result in oppressive sensations in the chest and abdomen and loss of appetite.

159	160	161

159
PANAX GINSENG
(Araliaceae)
GINSENG

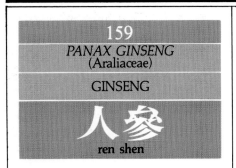

人參
ren shen

Natural distribution: Northeastern China, northern Korea
Parts used: Roots
Nature: Sweet; neutral
Affinity: Spleen, lungs
Effects: Very tonifying to primordial energy; tonic to lungs and spleen; nourishes vital fluids; aphrodisiac
Indications: Energy deficiency: weak pulse, asthma due to "empty" lungs, dyspepsia, lack of appetite, prolapse of rectum, hypertension, insomnia, heart palpitations; diabetes
Dosage: Normal—2-8 g;
acute—15-20 g
Remarks: Strictly avoid tea and turnips when using ginseng; ginseng regulates blood pressure and blood sugar as well; promotes secretion of sexual hormones in men and women; promotes blood production by tonifying *qi*

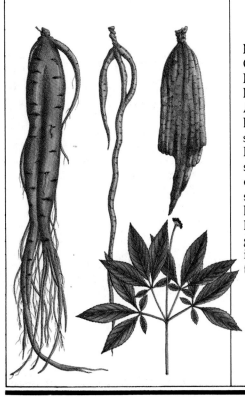

160
CODONOPSIS TANGSHEN
(Campanulaceae)

黨參
dang shen

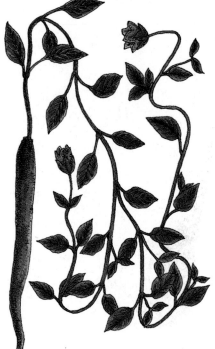

Natural distribution: Northern China
Parts used: Roots
Nature: Sweet, warm
Affinity: Spleen, lungs
Effects: Tonic to spleen and lungs; stomachic
Indications: Energy deficiency: fatigue, shallow and strained breathing, lack of appetite, dyspepsia, facial swelling, prolapse of rectum
Dosage: 10-15 g
Remarks: Similar in action to ginseng, but not as strong; this drug is often substituted in places or at times when ginseng is too expensive

161
ASTRAGALUS MEMBRANACEUS
(Leguminosae)

黃蓍
huang qi

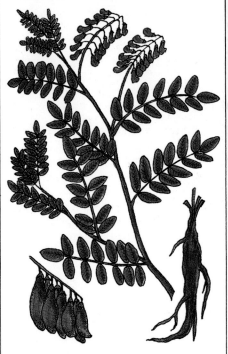

Natural distribution: Northern China, Mongolia, Manchuria
Parts used: Roots
Nature: Sweet; slightly warm
Affinity: Spleen, lungs
Effects: Tonifies energy; diuretic; impedes perspiration; promotes suppuration of abscesses
Indications: Energy deficiency: fatigue, prolapse of rectum, womb, or other organs; profuse sweating due to external "empty" ailments; stubborn abscesses; facial swelling; diabetes
Dosage: 8-15 g
Remarks: The drug is also cardiotonic, and lowers blood pressure and blood sugar; improves circulation in flesh and skin

144

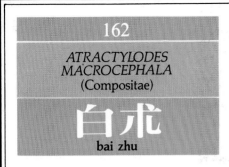

162
ATRACTYLODES MACROCEPHALA (Compositae)

白朮
bai zhu

Natural distribution: China, Korea, Japan
Parts used: Roots
Nature: Sweet and bitter; warm
Affinity: Spleen, stomach
Effects: Tonic to spleen; drying; diuretic; impedes perspiration
Indications: "Empty" stomach and spleen: full feeling after small food intake, fatigue, diarrhoea; phlegm and swelling due to damp-excess; profuse perspiration due to "empty-cold" ailments
Dosage: 3-10 g
Remarks: The drug is sedative to restless foetus

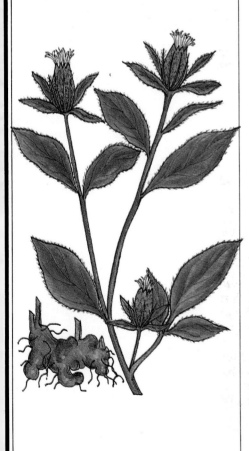

163
DIOSCOREA OPPOSITA (Dioscoreaceae)
CHINESE YAM

山藥
shan yao

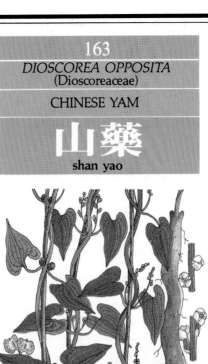

Natural distribution: China, Japan
Parts used: Roots (tubers)
Nature: Sweet; neutral
Affinity: Spleen, lungs
Effects: Tonic to spleen, stomach, and lungs; stomachic; digestive
Indications: "Empty" spleen and stomach: lack of appetite, fatigue, diarrhoea, leukorrhoea; chronic coughs; nocturnal emissions; spermatorrhoea; frequent and scanty urination
Dosage: 10-30 g
Remarks: The drug also lowers blood-sugar and is used in diabetes

164
ZIZIPHUS JUJUBA (Rhamnaceae)
CHINESE JUJUBE (cultivated variety)

大棗
da zao

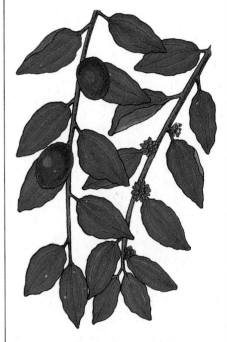

Natural distribution: China, Japan, India, Afghanistan
Parts used: Fruits
Nature: Sweet; neutral
Affinity: Spleen
Effects: Tonic to spleen and stomach; nutrient; sedative
Indications: "Empty" spleen and stomach; general energy deficiency; fatigue; hysteria
Dosage: 3-5 fruits
Remarks: The plant is added to many strong tonic prescriptions as a metabolic buffer to slow down and prolong their effects

165
GLYCYRRHIZA URALENSIS (Leguminosae)
CHINESE LICORICE

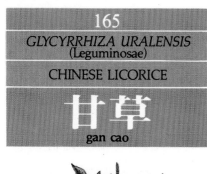

甘草

gan cao

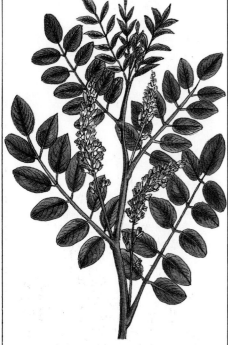

Natural distribution: Northern China, Mongolia, Siberia

Parts used: Roots

Nature: Sweet; neutral

Affinity: Enters all 12 meridians and organs

Effects: Tonic; antipyretic; antidote; demulcent to lungs; expectorant; analgesic

Indications: "Empty" spleen and stomach; blood and energy deficiency; toxic abscesses; swollen and sore throat; coughs; asthma; acute abdominal pains

Dosage: 2-10 g

Remarks: This is the most commonly used Chinese herb, appearing in almost all prescriptions; it benefits all the organs; its flavour improves the taste of all prescriptions; it slows and prolongs the effects of strong tonic prescriptions; antidote in mushroom poisoning; emollient in peptic ulcers

166
DRIED HUMAN PLACENTA

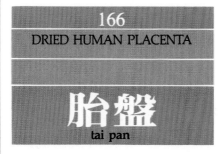

胎盤

tai pan

Natural distribution: World-wide

Parts used: Dried placenta tissue

Nature: Sweet and salty; warm

Affinity: Heart, spleen, kidneys

Effects: Tonifies energy, blood, and vital essence

Indications: Extreme blood and energy deficiency; general weakness and fatigue; asthma due to lung deficiency

Dosage: 3-5 g

Remarks: Also an effective tonic in impotence, sterility and neurasthenia

YANG-TONICS

Yang-tonics are used in ailments caused by yang-deficiency. The kidneys house primordial yang-energy, and thus most yang-deficient ailments come to rest in the kidneys, and yang-tonics primarily tonify and "warm" that organ. Common symptoms of kidney-yang deficiency are fear of cold, cold hands and feet, impotence, spermatorrhoea, nocturnal emissions, premature ejaculation, urinal incontinence, etc. Sexual potency falls within the domain of yang and also centres about the kidneys and surrounding glands. Thus, the most renowned Chinese aphrodisiacs fall into the yang-tonic category. Aphrodisiac tonics, however, should only be used in cases of yang-deficiency. If used by people with yang-excess and/or yin-deficiency, they further aggravate the yin/yang imbalance by injuring the already weak yin-energy.

The other organs affected by yang-deficiency are the spleen and the heart. Spleen-yang deficient ailments are similar to those of "spleen-empty", described above under "Energy Tonics". Heart-yang deficiencies, which display symptoms of profuse cold sweats, pale complexion, and weak, irregular pulse, are injurious to the blood and circulation and are best treated with drugs which "warm" the blood and with energy tonics. The liver and lungs rarely display yang-deficient ailments: on the contrary, yang-excess is the most common imbalance in those two organs.

Yang-tonics are generally warm and drying and should be used sparingly by patients with chronic yin-deficiency or fire-excess.

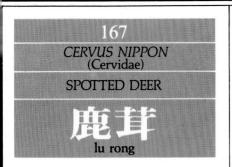

167

CERVUS NIPPON
(Cervidae)

SPOTTED DEER

鹿茸

lu rong

Natural distribution: Northeastern China, northwestern China
Parts used: Horn, velvet antler
Nature: Sweet and salty; warm
Affinity: Liver, kidneys
Effects: Tonic to kidney-yang; tonic to the 13th and 14th meridians (meridians of "Life" and of "Conception"); nutrient tonic to semen, marrow, sinew, and cartilage; aphrodisiac
Indications: Kidney-yang deficiency (insufficient secretions of sexual hormones): impotence, watery semen, cold extremities, lumbago, clear and profuse urine, anemia, weight loss, slow growth in children, weak bone and sinews, dysmennorhoea, leukorrhoea; 13th and 14th meridian deficiencies
Dosage: Pure powder—0.3-1 g; decoction—3-5 g
Remarks: This is one of the most renowned and popular sexual tonics in the *ben cao*; the best is tender new horn still in velvet with the dried blood still visible in the cartilage; the most potent essence is obtained by drinking the fresh blood and secretions directly from the freshly cut horn

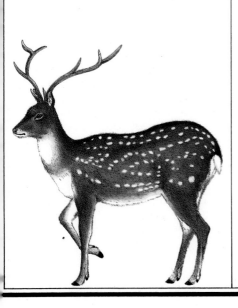

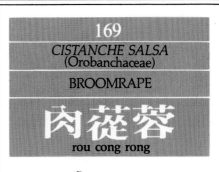

168

EPIMEDIUM SAGITTATUM
(Berberidaceae)

HORNY GOAT WEED

淫羊藿

yin yang huo

Natural distribution: China, Japan
Parts used: Leaves
Nature: Pungent; warm
Affinity: Liver, kidneys
Effects: Tonic to kidney-yang; eliminates "wind-damp" ailments (rheumatic); aphrodisiac
Indications: Kidney-yang deficiency: impotence, spermatorrhoea, premature ejaculation, lumbago, cold hands and feet, fear of cold; rheumatic discomforts of "wind-damp" excess; spasms; numbness
Dosage: 10-15 g
Remarks: The drug dilates the capillaries and larger blood vessels; lowers blood pressure; common ingredient in "Spring Wine"; remedies absent-mindedness by flooding the brain with blood

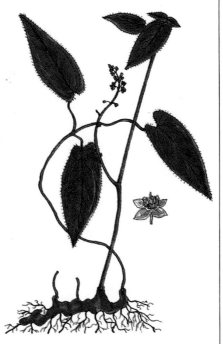

169

CISTANCHE SALSA
(Orobanchaceae)

BROOMRAPE

肉蓯蓉

rou cong rong

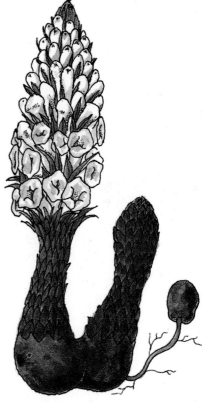

Natural distribution: Northern China, Mongolia, Siberia
Parts used: Fleshy stems
Nature: Sweet and salty; warm
Affinity: Kidneys, large intestine
Effects: Tonic to kidney-yang; demulcent laxative; aphrodisiac
Indications: Kidney-yang deficiency: impotence, spermatorrhoea; premature ejaculation, lumbago, weak bones and sinews; constipation due to dry intestines
Dosage: 10-15 g
Remarks: Tonifies yin as well as yang; lowers blood pressure

170

ALPINIA OXYPHYLLA
(Zingiberaceae)

BLACK CARDAMON

益智仁
yi zhi ren

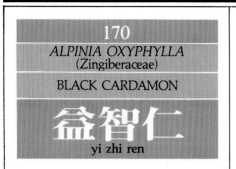

Natural distribution: Southern China
Parts used: Seeds
Nature: Pungent; warm
Affinity: Spleen, kidneys
Effects: Tonic to kidney-yang; nutrient to bones and sinew; inhibits excess urination; antidiarrhoeic; astringent; stomachic
Indications: Kidney-yang deficiency: impotence, premature ejaculation, frequent and profuse urination, urinal incontinence; "cold" spleen symptoms: diarrhoea, profuse salivation, cold and pain in abdomen
Dosage: 3-10 g

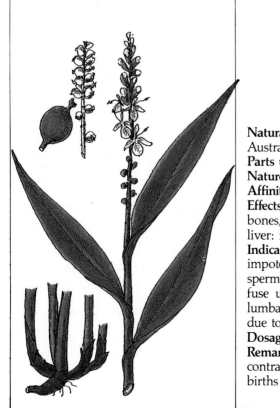

171

TRIBULUS TERRESTRIS
(Zygophylaceae)

CALTROP

刺蒺藜
ci ji li

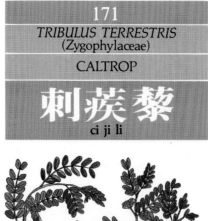

Natural distribution: China, Australia, Africa, South America
Parts used: Mature fruits
Nature: Sweet; warm
Affinity: Liver, kidneys
Effects: Tonic to kidneys; nutrient to bones, sinew and cartilage; tonic to liver: improves vision
Indications: Kidney-yang deficiency: impotence, premature ejaculation, spermatorrhoea, frequent and profuse urination, ringing in the ears, lumbago, leukorrhoea; blurry vision due to liver deficiency
Dosage: 10-15 g
Remarks: The drug facilitates labour contractions during difficult childbirths

172

CUSCUTA JAPONICA
(Convulvulaceae)

DODDER

菟絲子
tu si zi

Natural distribution: China, Japan
Parts used: Seeds
Nature: Pungent and sweet; neutral
Affinity: Liver, kidneys
Effects: Tonic to kidneys; nutrient to bones, sinew and cartilage; tonic to liver: improves vision
Indications: Kidney deficiency: impotence, premature ejaculation, spermatorrhoea, ringing in ears, frequent and profuse urination, urinal incontinence, lumbago, leukorrhoea; blurry vision due to liver deficiency
Dosage: 10-15 g

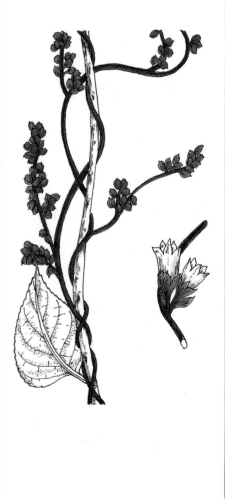

173
CNIDIUM MONNIERI
(Umbelliferae)

蛇床子

she chuang zi

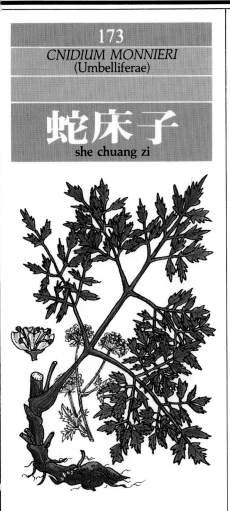

Natural distribution: China, Vietnam, Laos, eastern Europe
Parts used: Fruits
Nature: Pungent and bitter; warm
Affinity: Kidneys
Effects: Tonic to kidney-yang; anti-rheumatic; antiseptic; aphrodisiac; astringent; stimulant
Indications: Kidney-yang deficiency: especially impotence and female sterility; external application to vaginal itching and infections, abscesses and ringworm
Dosage: 5-10 g
Remarks: A decoction of this herb is a highly effective antiseptic wash for vaginal itching, yeast infections, parasites, etc.

174
DIPSACUS ASPER
(Dipsacaceae)

TEASEL

續斷

xu duan

Natural distribution: Central China
Parts used: Roots
Nature: Bitter; slightly warm
Affinity: Liver, kidneys
Effects: Tonic to kidneys and liver; nutrient to bones, sinew and cartilage; promotes muscle growth; hemostatic
Indications: Kidney deficiency; liver deficiency; lumbago; cold extremities; traumatic injury to bone and sinews; menorrhagia; bleeding during pregnancy
Dosage: 10-15 g
Remarks: Effective hemostatic action in female menstrual disorders; eliminates pus from abscesses and wounds

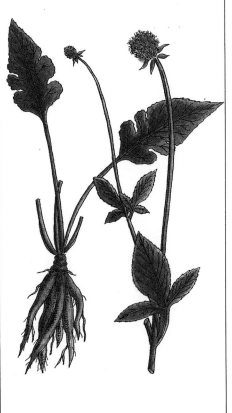

175
EUCOMMIA ULMOIDES
(Eucommiaceae)

EUCOMMIA

杜仲

du zhong

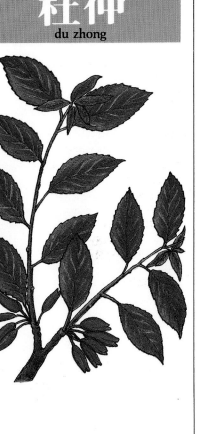

Natural distribution: Central China
Parts used: Bark
Nature: Sweet; warm
Affinity: Liver, kidneys
Effects: Tonic to liver and kidneys; nutrient to bone, sinew and cartilage; sedative to restless foetus
Indications: Kidney deficiency; liver deficiency; lumbago, dizziness; headaches; weakness and fatigue; impotence; frequent urination; weakness, dizziness restless foetus and lumbago in pregnant women
Dosage: 10-15 g
Remarks: The drug lowers blood pressure; preventive in miscarriage; an especially effective remedy for lumbago due to kidney deficiency

BLOOD TONICS

Blood tonics are used to "nourish the blood" in diseases caused by blood deficiency. Common symptoms of "empty" blood ailments are a sallow complexion, pale lips, colourless fingernails, dizziness, ringing in the ears, heart palpitations, absent-mindedness, insomnia, etc. Dysmenorrhoea is an additional symptom in women.

When blood deficiency appears together with energy deficiency, both energy and blood tonics should be applied in therapy. If yin-deficiency is also indicated, yin-tonics are used as well. Basically blood tonics and yin tonics have similar effects, the former being more specific to the blood and the latter generally affecting the entire body.

Blood tonics are generally moist and "sticky" by nature. Many have high oil and moisture content. Those patients suffering from stagnation, abdominal oppression, and poor appetite due to damp-excess should use them sparingly. If the spleen is "empty," combine blood tonics with stomachic and digestive herbs.

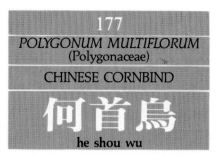

176
REHMANNIA GLUTINOSA
(Scrophulariaceae)

熟地黃
shu di huang

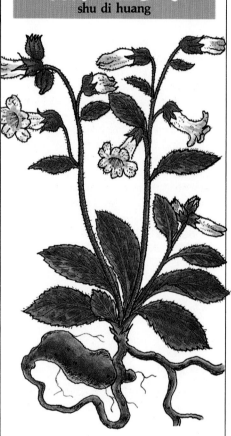

Natural distribution: Northern China
Parts used: Roots (steamed)
Nature: Sweet; slightly warm
Affinity: Heart, liver, kidneys
Effects: Tonic to blood; nourishes yin; hemostatic
Indications: Blood deficiency: dizziness, heart palpitations, insomnia, dysmenorrhoea; menorrhagia; kidney-yin deficiency: nocturnal sweats, spermatorrhoea, diabetes
Dosage: 10-30 g
Remarks: The fresh root is refrigerant to blood and nourishes yin (see Antipyretics, page 00); the steamed root is exclusively used to tonify blood and nourish yin

177
POLYGONUM MULTIFLORUM
(Polygonaceae)

CHINESE CORNBIND

何首烏
he shou wu

Natural distribution: Southwestern China, Japan, Taiwan
Parts used: Roots, stems and leaves
Nature: Bitter and sour; slightly warm
Affinity: Liver, kidneys
Effects: Tonic to liver and kidneys; nourishes blood and semen; demulcent laxative; antidote
Indications: Blood deficiency: sallow complexion, dizziness, insomnia, premature greying of hair; kidney deficiency: lumbago, weak bone, sinew and cartilage; constipation due to dry intestines; swelling of lymph glands; abscesses and ulcers
Dosage: 7-15 g
Remarks: Contemporary usage shows the drug to be effective against high blood pressure and hardening of the veins and arteries

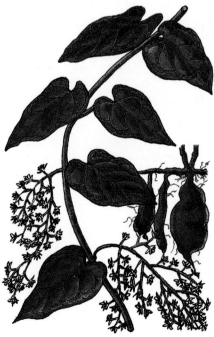

178
ANGELICA SINENSIS
(Umbelliferae)

當歸
dang gui

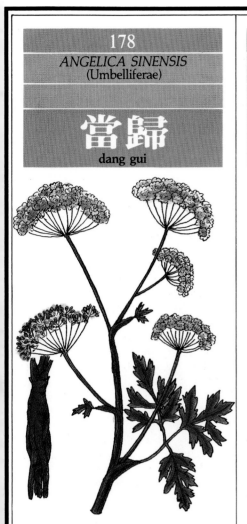

Natural distribution: Central China
Parts used: Roots
Nature: Sweet and pungent; warm
Affinity: Liver, spleen
Effects: Tonic to blood; emennagogue; promotes circulation; analgesic; sedative; laxative
Indications: Menstrual disorders: dysmenorrhoea, menorrhagia, amenorrhoea; blood deficiency: painful scarring in traumatic injuries, postnatal abdominal pain; rheumatic pains
Dosage: 10-15 g
Remarks: This is the most important drug for menstrual disorders

179
EQUUS ASINUS
(Equidae)
ASS-HIDE GLUE

阿膠
e jiao

Natural distribution: World-wide
Parts used: Glue prepared from the hides
Nature: Sweet; neutral
Affinity: Lungs, liver, kidneys
Effects: Tonic to blood; hemostatic; nourishes yin; demulcent to lungs
Indications: Blood deficiency: sallow complexion, dizziness, heart palpitations, blood in urine, stool, or sputum, menorrhagia; insomnia and restlessness of heat excess
Dosage: 10-15g

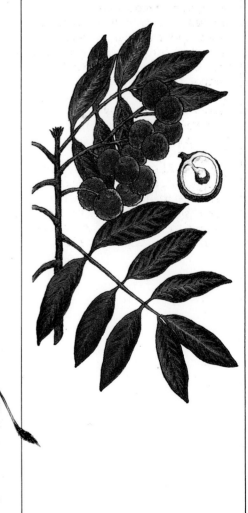

180
EUPHORIA LONGAN
(Sapindaceae)
LONGAN FRUIT

龍眼肉
long yan rou

Natural distribution: Southern China, Japan
Parts used: Dried flesh of the fruits
Nature: Sweet; warm
Affinity: Heart, spleen
Effects: Cardiotonic; sedative; tonic to blood: digestive
Indications: Heart and spleen deficiency; absent-mindedness; insomnia; heart palpitations; weakness, fatigue due to blood deficiency
Dosage: 10-15 g
Remarks: The kernels are ground to powder and applied as a styptic to abscesses, sores, wounds, etc.

YIN TONICS

Yin-tonics are applied in "yin-empty" ailments. They nourish kidney-yin, lung-yin, stomach-yin, and liver-yin and are used against ailments of deficiency ("empty") in those organs. Major symptoms of such ailments are as follows: (1) Lung-yin deficiency: dry coughs, blood in sputum, "empty" body-heat, thirst, irritability. (2) Stomach-yin deficiency: red lips, dark red tongue, peeling tongue fur, fluid deficiency, thirst, lack of hunger. (3) Liver-yin deficiency: dry eyes, blurry vision, dizziness, headaches. (4) Kidney-yin deficiency: afternoon heat spells, nocturnal sweats, spermatorrhoea.

Most yin-tonics are sweet, cold, moist, and "sticky" by nature. Patients with spleen-yang and kidney-yang deficiencies (for symptoms see "Yang Tonics") should use yin-tonics sparingly and in combination with other appropriate herbs.

181
ADENOPHORA TETRAPHYLLA
(Campanulaceae)

沙參
sha shen

Natural distribution: China, Japan
Parts used: Roots
Nature: Sweet; slightly cold
Affinity: Lungs, stomach
Effects: Demulcent to lungs; antitussive; stomachic; expectorant

Indications: Lung-yin deficiency: dry coughs, chronic coughs, body-heat, faint and feeble voice; stomach-yin deficiency: thirst, insufficient salivation, red lips
Dosage: 8-15 g

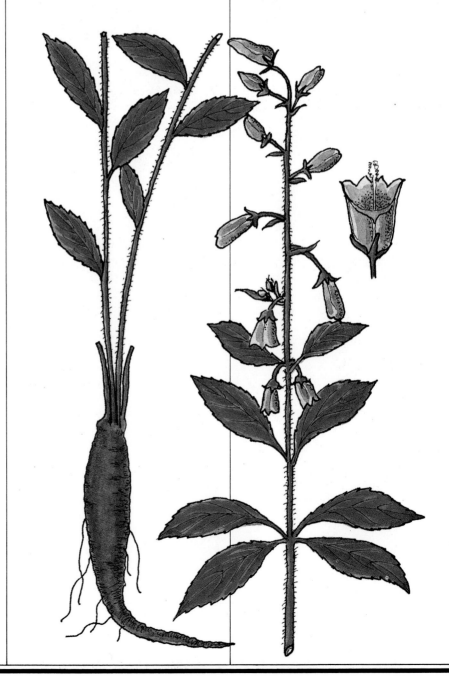

182
LIRIOPE SPICATA
(Liliaceae)

CREEPING LILY-TURF

麥門冬
mai men dong

Natural distribution: China, Japan
Parts used: Root-tubers
Nature: Sweet and slightly bitter; slightly cold
Affinity: Heart, lungs, stomach
Effects: Refrigerant to heart; demulcent to lungs; stomachic; emollient; antitussive
Indications: Lung-yin deficiency: dry coughs, blood in sputum, irritability; thirst due to fluid deficiency
Dosage: 4-10 g
Remarks: Promotes lactation

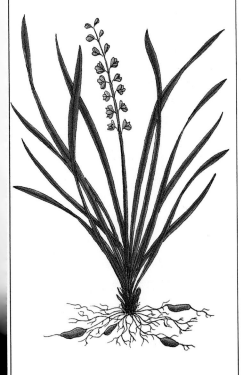

183
LYCIUM CHINENSE
(Solanaceae)

CHINESE WOLFBERRY

枸杞子
gou qi zi

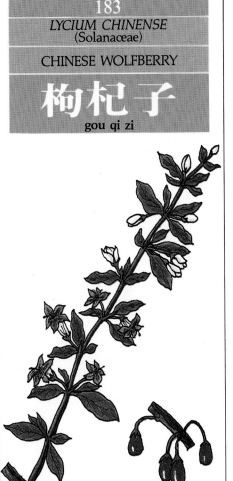

Natural distribution: China, Japan
Parts used: Fruits
Nature: Sweet; neutral
Affinity: Liver, kidneys
Effects: Tonic to kidneys: nourishes semen; tonic to liver: improves vision
Indications: Liver-yin deficiency: blurry vision, dizziness, headaches; kidney-yin deficiency: spermatorrhoea, lumbago
Dosage: 4-10 g
Remarks: The herb is also an effective remedy in mild forms of diabetes

184
ECLIPTA PROSTRATA
(Compositae)

旱蓮草
han lian cao

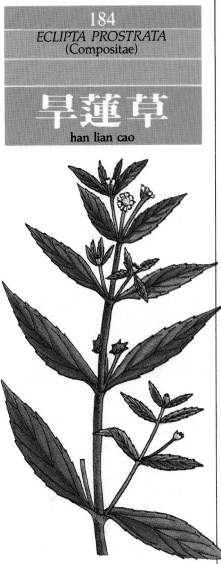

Natural distribution: China, Japan, Taiwan, Indochina
Parts used: Whole plant
Nature: Sweet and sour; cold
Affinity: Liver, kidneys
Effects: Tonic to yin; tonic to kidney-yin; refrigerant to blood; hemostatic; astringent
Indications: Liver-yin deficiency: blurry vision, dizziness, headache; kidney-yin deficiency: spermatorrhoea, premature greying of hair; bleeding due to yin-deficiency: blood in sputum, urine and bile, menorrhagia
Dosage: 10-15 g
Remarks: An extract of the fresh herb applied to the scalp promotes hair growth; taken internally, it blackens the hair, beard and eyebrows

185

CHINEMYS REEVESII
(Testudinidae)

TURTLE

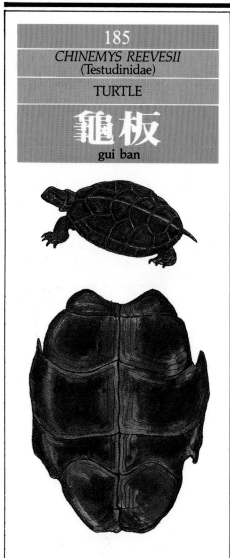

龜板

gui ban

Natural distribution: World-wide
Parts used: Lower shell (underside)
Nature: Salty and sweet; neutral
Affinity: Kidneys, heart, liver
Effects: Tonic to yin; tonic to kidneys; nutrient to sinew, bone and cartilage
Indications: Kidney-yin deficiency: faint and weak voice, afternoon heat spells, nocturnal sweats, lumbago, weak sinews, bone and cartilage; yin-deficiency due to heat injuries; failure of opening in top of baby's scull to close; menorrhagia
Dosage: 10-25 g
Remarks: Promotes contractions in delayed or difficult childbirth; promotes growth of bone and cartilage in babies

186

TRIONYX SINENSIS
(Trionychidae)

TORTOISE

鱉甲

bie jia

Natural distribution: World-wide
Parts used: Upper shell (topside)
Nature: Salty; neutral
Affinity: Liver, spleen, kidneys
Effects: Tonic to yin; clears blockages and softens tumours; antipyretic
Indications: Kidney-yin deficiency: afternoon heat spells, nocturnal sweats; yin-deficiency due to yang-excess; yin-deficiency due to heat excess; swollen or infected pancreas; pain in rib-cage; amenorrhoea; tumours
Dosage: 10-20 g

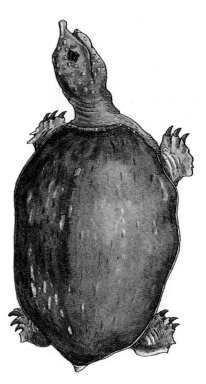

ASTRINGENT OR "WITHDRAW AND HOLD BACK"

Medicines which contract and tighten tissues to impede uncontrolled seepage of fluids are called "astringent". They are employed in ailments of fluid loss with such symptoms as profuse sweating, nocturnal sweats, chronic diarrhoea and dysentery, chronic coughs, spermatorrhoea, premature ejaculation, urinal incontinence, chronic leukorrhoea, profuse bleeding, etc. Chronic fluid loss is harmful to the body's primordial energies, and if left unchecked, it can lead to far more serious, acute ailments.

The primary pharmacodynamic effects of astringents are to impede perspiration, stop diarrhoea, strengthen and "solidify" the semen, retain urine, stop leukorrhoea, hemostatic, antitussive, and other fluid preserving actions. In cases of external and "full" ailments which have not been fully eliminated, and in the early stages of dysentery and hacking coughs, astringents should not be used, in order to prevent retention of "evil-*qi*" excess.

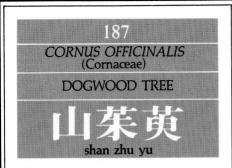

187
CORNUS OFFICINALIS
(Cornaceae)

DOGWOOD TREE

山茱萸
shan zhu yu

Natural distribution: Eastern China, Korea, Japan
Parts used: Fruits
Nature: Sour; slightly warm
Affinity: Liver, kidneys
Effects: Tonic to liver and kidneys; astringent; hemostatic
Indications: Kidney deficiency: impotence, spermatorrhoea, premature ejaculation, lumbago vertigo, nocturnal sweats, urinal incontinence; liver deficiency: dizziness, blurry vision, headaches
Dosage: 5-10 g

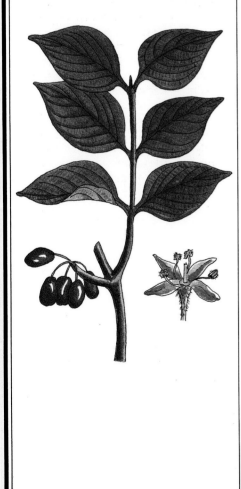

188
SCHISANDRA CHINENSIS
(Magnoliaceae)

SCHISANDRA

五味子
wu wei zi

Natural distribution: Northeastern China, Manchuria, Japan
Parts used: Dried berries
Nature: Sour; warm
Affinity: Lungs, kidneys
Effects: Astringent; tonic to kidneys; demulcent; antidiarrhoeic; antitussive
Indications: Chronic coughs; asthma; thirst; profuse perspiration due to "empty" ailments; spermatorrhoea; nocturnal emissions; profuse and frequent urination; chronic diarrhoea
Dosage: 2-5 g
Remarks: The drug is both astringent and demulcent, depending on the condition of the patient's fluid balance: in cases of fluid excess, it dries; in cases of fluid deficiency, it moistens

189
TERMINALIA CHEBULA
(Combretaceae)

MYROBALAN

訶子
he zi

Natural distribution: Indochina, Malaysia
Parts used: Fruits
Nature: Bitter and sour; neutral
Affinity: Lungs, large intestine
Effects: Astringent, antidiarrhoeic; hemostatic
Indications: Chronic diarrhoea and dysentery; prolapse of rectum; asthma and coughs due to "empty" lungs; leukorrhoea; menorrhagia
Dosage: 3-8 g
Remarks: The drug is highly astringent, especially in the large intestine

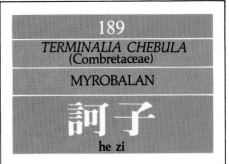

190	191	192
RHUS CHINENSIS (Anacardiaceae)	*PAPAVER SOMNIFERUM* (Papaveraceae)	*EURYALE FEROX* (Nymphaeaceae)
CHINESE NUT-GALL TREE	OPIUM POPPY	FOXNUT
五倍子	罌粟殻	芡實
wu bei zi	ying su ke	qian shi

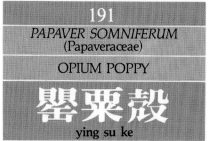

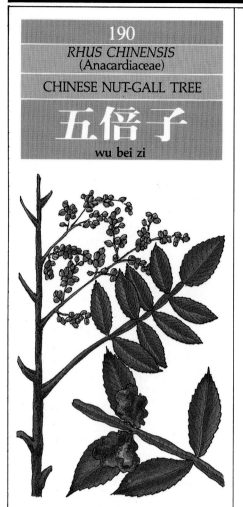

Natural distribution: China, India, Mediterranean
Parts used: The dried empty capsules from which the opium latex has already been extracted
Nature: Sour; neutral
Affinity: Lungs, large intestine, kidneys
Effects: Astringent to lungs and large intestine; analgesic; antitussive
Indications: Chronic cough; chronic diarrhoea and dysentery; stomach ache; prolapse of rectum; asthma; opium withdrawal
Dosage: 4-10 g
Remarks: The extracted opium is also used in medicine: its action is narcotic, sedative, hypnotic, antispasmodic, astringent and analgesic

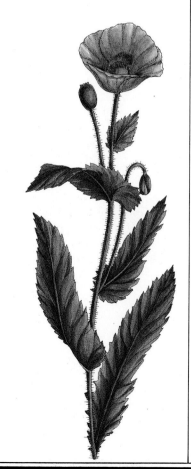

Natural distribution: China, Japan, India
Parts used: Seeds
Nature: Sweet and sour; neutral
Affinity: Spleen, kidneys
Effects: Astringent; analgesic; tonic to kidneys and spleen
Indications: Kidney deficiency: spermatorrhoea, impotence, premature ejaculation, nocturnal emissions, urinal incontinence; spleen deficiency: chronic diarrhoea, dyspepsia; leukorrhoea due to damp excess
Dosage: 10-30 g

Natural distribution: China
Parts used: Hard, globular excretions on the leaves and stems induced by the larva deposited there by the aphid insect *Melaphis chinensis*
Nature: Sour; cold
Affinity: Lungs, kidneys, large intestine
Effects: Astringent to lungs and large intestine; antipyretic; hemostatic
Indications: Chronic coughs; chronic diarrhoea and dysentery; profuse perspiration due to "empty" ailments; bleeding hemorrhoids and stools; spermatorrhoea
Dosage: 1-3 g
Remarks: The drug has highly astringent action; contains 70% tannin

193	194	195
PARATENODERA SINENSIS (Mantidae)	*RUBUS COREANUS* (Rosaceae)	*SEPIA ESCULENTA* (Sepiidae)
PRAYING MANTIS	BLACKBERRY	CUTTLEFISH
桑螵蛸	覆盆子	海螵蛸
sang piao xiao	fu pen zi	hai piao xiao

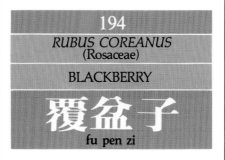

Natural distribution: World-wide
Parts used: Eggcase
Nature: Sweet and salty; neutral
Affinity: Liver, kidneys
Effects: Tonic to kidney-yang; astringent
Indications: Kidney-yang deficiency: impotence, spermatorrhoea, premature ejaculation, urinal incontinence, bed-wetting
Dosage: 3-10 g

Natural distribution: Central China, Europe
Parts used: Unripe berries
Nature: Sweet and sour; slightly warm
Affinity: Liver, kidneys
Effects: Tonic to kidneys; astringent
Indications: Kidney deficiency: impotence, spermatorrhoea, premature ejaculation, urinal incontinence, bed-wetting
Dosage: 5-10 g
Remarks: The drug improves vision in liver and kidney deficient symptoms

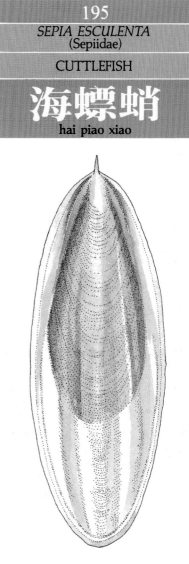

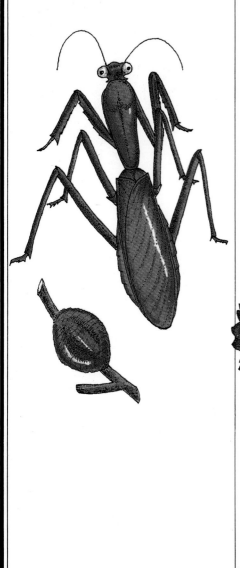

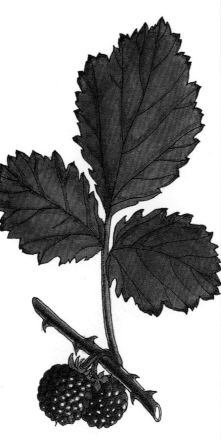

Natural distribution: World-wide
Parts used: Cuttlefish bone
Nature: Salty; slightly warm
Affinity: Liver, kidneys
Effects: Astringent; hemostatic; neutralizes stomach acid; styptic to abscesses and sores
Indications: Menorrhagia; bleeding abscesses, sores and wounds; spermatorrhoea; leukorrhoea; stomach ulcers; rising bile; pruritis
Dosage: 4-10 g
Remarks: Highly astringent: prolonged or excess use may induce constipation

ANTHELMINTIC OR "DRIVE OUT WORMS"

Drugs which kill or expel intestinal worms are called "anthelmintic." Worms enter the body through the skin or as ova in contaminated foods. Some can only be detected by examining the faeces for ova. Other types are indicated by such symptoms as abdominal pain and pressure, loss of weight, loss of appetite, eating without satisfying hunger, desire for strange foods or materials, yellow complexion, body swelling, and itchy anus. Treatment of intestinal worms should always be followed up with appropriate preventive care to prevent recurrence of contamination.

Anthelmintic herbs should be used with the following points in mind:

— Prolonged worm infestation with attendant symptoms of abdominal stagnation should be treated in combination with digestives.
— Anthelmintics are most effectively administered on an empty stomach, to insure direct contact with the worms. If patients also suffer from chronic constipation, combine treatment with cathartics or laxatives to insure thorough elimination of worms and their ova.
— Dosages of anthelmintics should be carefully regulated, especially with highly poisonous herbs, to prevent toxification
— When fever or acute abdominal pain is displayed, use of anthelmintics should be temporarily halted
— These drugs should be used sparingly in pregnant women, the weak, and the elderly.

196
QUISQUALIS INDICA
(Combretaceae)

RANGOON CREEPER

使君子
shi jun zi

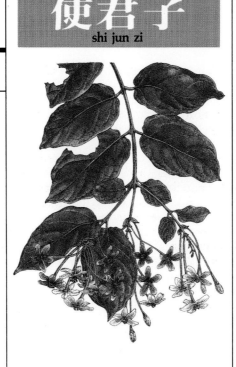

Natural distribution: Southern China, India, Indochina
Parts used: Fruits
Nature: Sweet; warm
Affinity: Spleen, stomach
Effects: Anthelmintic; digestive
Indications: Pains and pressure in abdomen due to stagnation caused by tapeworms; abdominal swelling and swollen limbs in children due to intestinal parasites
Dosage: 4-8 g (1 fruit per year of age in children)
Remarks: This is an important drug in treating parasitic contamination in children

---

197
ARECA CATECHU
(Palmae)

BETEL PALM

檳榔
bing lang

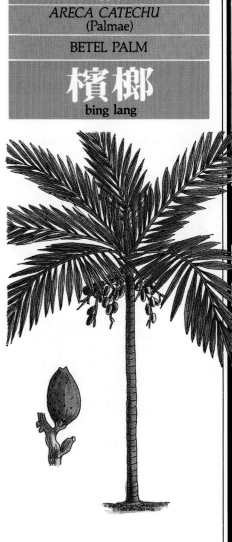

Natural distribution: Indochina, India, Taiwan
Parts used: Betel Nuts
Nature: Pungent and bitter; warm
Affinity: Stomach, large intestine
Effects: Anthelmintic; digestive; diuretic
Indications: All types of intestinal worms; stagnant accumulations of undigested food; irregular bowel movements; swelling in feet and legs
Dosage: 4-10 g
Remarks: Also used in malaria

198	199	200
CUCURBITA MOSCHATA (Cucurbitaceae) PUMPKIN # 南瓜子 nan gua zi	*DRYOPTERIS CRASSIRHIZOMA* (Dryopteridaceae) # 貫衆 guan zhong	*ALLIUM SATIVUM* (Liliaceae) GARLIC # 大蒜 da suan

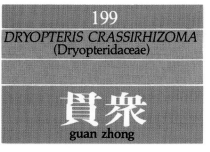

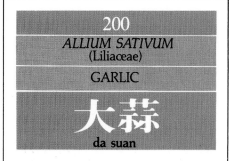

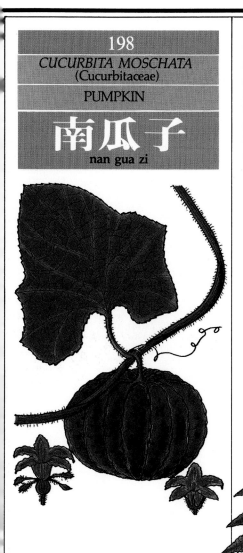

Natural distribution: World-wide
Parts used: Rhizomes
Nature: Bitter; slightly cold
Affinity: Liver, stomach
Effects: Anthelmintic; antipyretic; antidote; hemostatic
Indications: All types of intestinal worms; pain and pressure in abdomen; inflamed and infected abscesses due to heat excess; thyroid inflammations; menorrhagia
Dosage: 8-15 g
Remarks: Mildly poisonous; effective preventive against contagious colds

Natural distribution: World-wide
Parts used: Bulbs
Nature: Pungent, warm
Affinity: Stomach, large intestine
Effects: Anthelmintic; antiseptic; antidote; stomachic; tonic
Indications: Hookworm, pinworm; diarrhoea and dysentery; tuberculosis; coughing fits; external application to early stages of abscesses and ringworm on the head
Dosage: 3-5 cloves (fresh)
Remarks: Extracts of this family of herbs have recently become popular remedies in the West; it has been often noted that countries which consume large quantities of garlic have a lower incidence of cancer than others; the herb is by far more effective when used fresh

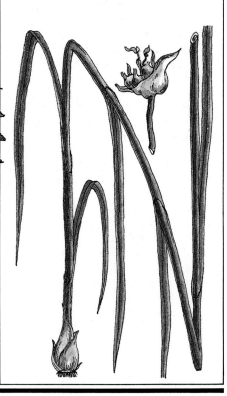

Natural distribution: World-wide
Parts used: Seeds
Nature: Sweet; warm
Affinity: (Natural affinities not determined)
Effects: Anthelmintic
Indications: Intestinal worms; swelling and pain in abdomen
Dosage: 30-50 g
Remarks: The herb is relatively new in Chinese medicine, which is why its affinities have not yet been established; usually followed up with cathartics

Herbal Prescriptions

The following herbal prescriptions have been taken from traditional Chinese herbal manuals and are representative of the various types of herbal remedies prepared for common ailments. They are effective against the ailments which fall within the normal bounds of their category. People with acute or highly complicated illnesses should consult qualified Chinese doctors to obtain herbal remedies for their specific problems.

The prescriptions have been divided into the three broad categories of Preventive, Curative, and Tonic. Various examples of each type are given according to the type of disease they cure.

The herbs are listed by their Latin botanical names and their reference numbers in this book are given in parentheses. Those with no number do not appear in the preceding list of 200 medicines, but are commonly available. The Chinese name in Chinese characters is also provided to facilitate filling the prescriptions at Chinese herb shops. Proportions and ingredients are in metric grams.

Generally, prescriptions which are prepared by decoction should be boiled in a covered earthenware or ceramic vessel over a low flame. If you find the taste unpleasant, a little sugar or honey may be added to improve the taste. One day's dosage is prepared at a time, usually divided into two or three portions. It is always best to consume herbal brews the same day they are prepared.

Preventive Prescriptions

CONTAGIOUS COLDS

Dryopteris crassizhizoma (199)

[貫眾]

6 months—2 years	3g
3 years —6 years	5g
7 years —10 years	7g
over 10 years	10g

Preparation
Boil with 3 cups water in covered earthen or ceramic vessel until it decocts to 1½ cups. Low fire. Strain through cheesecloth and take in 2 doses on empty stomach. Take 4 to 5 days during contagious season.

Remarks
Curative remedy in "wind-heat" ailments.

Lonicera japonica (47)   6g [金銀花]
Chrysanthemum morifolium (14)
                6g [菊花]
Euphoria longan (leaves) (180)
                4g [龍眼葉]

Preparation
Boil with 4 cups water in covered vessel until it decocts to 2-3 cups. Low fire. Strain through cheesecloth. Sweeten with sugar or honey. Drink through the day as tea.

Remarks
Curative remedy in "wind-heat" ailments.

Elsholtzia splendens (8)
                10g [香薷]

Preparation
Boil with 3 cups water in covered vessel until it decocts to 1½ cups. Strain. Drink as tea.

Remarks
Curative remedy in "wind-heat" ailments.

Allium fistulosum (9)
     4-5 stalks and rootlets [葱白]
Zingiber officinale (93) 20g [乾薑]
Raw sugar   to taste

Preparation
Boil with 3 cups water in covered vessel until it decocts to 2½ cups. Strain. Drink hot in 2 doses during the day on empty stomach.

Remarks
Curative remedy in "wind-heat" ailments.

MUMPS (Parotitis)

Baphicacanthus cusia   50g [板藍根]
Lonicera japonica (47)   20g [金銀花]

Preparation
Boil with 5 cups water in covered vessel until it decocts to 3 cups. Strain. Drink through the day. 4-5 days.

MENINGITIS

Phyllostachys (33)   20g [竹葉]
Gypsum fibrosum (29) 30g [石膏]

Preparation
Boil with 5 cups water in covered vessel until it decocts to 2½ cups. Strain. Drink on empty stomach in two doses per day. Let cool first. Use 4-5 days during contagious season.

ENCEPHALITIS

Baphicacanthus cusia   30g [板藍根]
Isatis tinctoria (44)   20g [大青葉]

Preparation
Boil with 5 cups water in covered vessel until it decocts to 3 cups. Strain. Drink through the day for 4-5 days as tea.

HEPATITIS

Artemisia capillaris (77)
                20g [茵陳蒿]
Ziziphus jujuba (164)
                7-8 pieces [大棗]

Preparation
Boil with 4 cups water in covered vessel until it decocts to 2 cups. Strain. Drink through the day as tea daily during contagious season.

HEAT-STROKE

Phyllostachys (33)   10g [竹葉]
Gypsum fibrosum (29) 10g [石膏]
Gardenia jasminoides (31)
                10g [梔子]
Lonicera japonica (47) 10g [金銀花]
Crataegus pinnatifida (138)
                10g [山楂]
Glycyrrhiza uralensis (165)
                10g [甘草]

Preparation
Boil with 4 cups water in covered vessel until it decocts to 2 cups. Strain. Drink through the day as tea.

Curative Prescriptions

HIGH BLOOD-PRESSURE

Lonicera japonica (47)   30g [金銀花]
Chrysanthemum morifolium (14)
　　　　　　　　30g [菊花]
Morus alba (13)   12g [桑葉]
Crataegus pinnatifida (138)
　　　　　　　　20g [山揸]
Cirsium japonicum (131)
　　　　　　　　20g [大薊]

Preparation
Boil with 5 cups water in covered vessel until it decocts to 3 cups. Strain. Take in 2 doses per day on empty stomach.

Gastrodia elata (109)   10g [天麻]
Uncaria rhynchophylla (110)
　　　　　　　　10g [鈎藤]
Haliotis gigantea (108)   20g [石決明]
Eucommia ulmoides (175)
　　　　　　　　20g [杜仲]
Loranthus yadoriki   10g [桑寄生]
Achyranthes bidentata (124)
　　　　　　　　10g [牛膝]
Gardenia jasminoides (31)
　　　　　　　　10g [梔子]
Scutellaria baicalensis (60)
　　　　　　　　10g [黃芩]
Leonurus artemisia   10g [益母草]
Polygonum multiflorum (vines) (177)
　　　　　　　　10g [何首烏]
Poria cocos (73)   10g [茯苓]

Preparation
Boil with 5 cups water in covered vessel until it decocts to 2 cups. Strain. Take in 2 doses per day on empty stomach.

CONSTIPATION

Indications
"Full-hot" type; fullness and pressure in abdomen; hot, foul breath; foul flatulence; hot feelings; thick, yellow tongue fur; headaches.

Rheum officinale (19)   6g [大黃]
Poncirus trifoliata (116)
　　　　　　　　10g [枳實]
Mirabilite (20)   10g [芒硝]
Magnolia officinalis (71)
　　　　　　　　10g [厚朴]

Preparation
Boil 2nd and 3rd ingredients with 3 cups water in covered vessel until it decocts to 1½ cups. Add first ingredient and boil 15 more minutes. Then add last ingredient and stir it in. Strain. Divide into 3 doses. If bowels do not move after first, take second, etc.

Indications
"Empty-cold" type; common in weak or elderly; desire to evacuate bowels without energy to do so; thin, pallid tongue fur; insomnia.

Codonopsis tangshen (160)
　　　　　　　　30g [黨參]
Astragalus membranaceus (161)
　　　　　　　　15g [黃蓍]
Cistanche salsa (169)   15g [肉蓯蓉]
Angelica sinensis (178)   10g [當歸]
Cannabis sativa (seeds) (23)
　　　　　　　　10g [火麻仁]

If insomnia is one of the symptoms, add the following:
Ziziphus jujuba (104)   15g [酸棗仁]
Thuja orientalis (seeds) (132)
　　　　　　　　10g [側柏葉]

Preparation
Boil with 5 cups water in covered vessel until it decocts to 3 cups. Strain. Divide into 2 doses and drink on empty stomach.

Indications
"Dry" type; pain and pressure in head; dry nose; thirst with desire for water; cracked, dry lips; hot palms and soles; chronic constipation; common in elderly and yin-deficient persons; sometimes occurs in women after childbirth.

Rehmannia glutinosa (38)
　　　　　　　　30g [乾地黃]
Scrophularia ningpoensis (45)
　　　　　　　　12g [玄參]
Liriope spicata (182)   10g [麥門冬]
Anemarrhena asphodeloides (30)
　　　　　　　　8g [知母]
Cannabis sativa (seeds) (23)
　　　　　　　　10g [火麻仁]
Trichosanthes kirilowii (roots)
　　　　　　　　10g [瓜蔞]
Trichosanthes kirilowii (seeds)
　　　　　　　　10g [天花粉]

If respiratory difficulties are among the symptoms, then add:
Codonopsis tangshen (160)
　　　　　　　　15g [黨參]
Atractylodes macrocephala (162)
　　　　　　　　10g [白朮]
If blood deficiency is indicated among the symptoms, then add:
Angelica sinensis (178)   12g [當歸]
Ligustrum lucidum (seeds)
　　　　　　　　10g [女貞子]

Preparation
Boil with 5 cups water in covered vessel until it decocts to 2 cups or less. Strain. Add honey 30-40 g. Take in 2 doses on empty stomach.

ACNE, PIMPLES

Schizonepeta tenuifolia (4)
　　　　　　　　8g [荊芥]
ledebouriella seseloides (5)
　　　　　　　　8g [防風]
Angelica anomala (7)   8g [白芷]
Bupleurum falcatum (16)
　　　　　　　　8g [柴胡]
Gardenia jasminoides (31)
　　　　　　　　8g [梔子]
Paeonia lactiflora (43)   8g [芍藥]
Forsythia suspensa (48)   8g [連翹]
Scutellaria baicalensis (60)
　　　　　　　　8g [黃芩]
Poncirus trifoliata (rind) (116)
　　　　　　　　8g [枳實]
Ligusticum wallichii (121)
　　　　　　　　8g [川芎]
Platycodon grandiflorum (144)
　　　　　　　　8g [桔梗]
Angelica sinensis (178)   8g [當歸]
Glycyrrhiza uralensis (165)
　　　　　　　　8g [甘草]

Preparation
Boil with 5 cups water in covered vessel until it decocts to 3 cups. Strain. Take in 2 doses per day on empty stomach. Avoid "pungent" and "hot" foods.

TOOTHACHE

Asarum sieboldii (6)   3g [細辛]
Rheum officinale (19)   5g [大黃]
Gypsum fibrosum (29)   20g [石膏]
Gardenia jasminoides (31)
　　　　　　　　10g [梔子]
Paeonia lactiflora (43)   6g [芍藥]
Scrophularia ningpoensis (45)
　　　　　　　　10g [玄參]
Prunus mume   3g

Preparation

First boil #29 for ½ hour on low fire with 4 cups water in covered vessel. Then add all other ingredients except #19. Decoct to 1½ cups, more or less. Then add #19 and continue to simmer for 15 min. Strain. Cool and take in 1 dose.

INDIGESTION due to excess consumption of meats and fats

Crataegus pinnatifida (138)
15g [山楂]
Citrus reticulata (115)   6g [陳皮]
Poncirus trifoliata (116) 8g [枳實]
Coptis sinensis (59)   4g [黃連]

Preparation

Boil with 3 cups water in covered vessel until it decocts to 1 cup. Strain. Take as one dose, sipping the brew gradually.

NERVOUS DISORDERS

Hysteria, irritability, hypertension, epilepsy, manic depression, violent temper, etc.
Glycyrrhiza uralensis (165)
12g [甘草]
Triticum aestivum (106)
30g [小麥]
Ziziphus jujuba (164)
10pieces [大棗]

Preparation

Boil with 3 cups water in covered vessel until it decocts to 1 cup. Strain. Take as one dose, sipping gradually.

FROST-BITE

Cinnamomum cassia (2)
10g [桂枝]
Paeonia lactiflora (43) 10g [芍藥]
Angelica sinensis (178) 12g [當歸]
Glycyrrhiza uralensis (165)
5g [甘草]
Ziziphus jujuba (164)
10 pieces [大棗]
Zingiber officinale (93) 5g [乾薑]

Preparation

Boil with 4 cups water in covered vessel until it decocts to 1½ cups, more or less. Strain. Take as 2 doses per day on empty stomach for about 1 week.

DYSMENORRHOEA

Saussurea lappa (117)   3g [木香]
Cyperus rotundus (118) 6g [香附]
Foeniculum vulgare (96) 2g [茴香]
Paeonia lactiflora (43)   6g [芍藥]
Curcuma aromatica (127)
6g [郁金]
Angelica sinensis (178) 10g [當歸]
Melia azedarach (seeds) 6g [川楝子]
Corydalis ambigua   6g [延胡索]
Citrus medica   3g [佛手柑]

If symptoms include pain and swelling of breasts, then add:
Bupleurum falcatum (16)
3g [柴胡]
Poncirus trifoliata (rind) (116)
6g [枳殼]
#43, #178 additional   6g each

If symptoms include constipation and dark, hot urine, then add:
Trichosanthes kirilowii (149)
12g [瓜蔞]
Plantago asiatica (75) 10g [車前子]
Areca catechu (197)   5g [檳榔]
Citrus reticulata (115)   6g [橘皮]

Preparation

Boil with 4 cups water in covered vessel until it decocts to 1½ cups. Strain. Take as two doses per day on empty stomach the first day pain begins.

PHLEGM

Excess accumulations of phlegm; hard phlegm lodged in the throat

Platycodon grandiflorum (144)
20g [桔梗]
Polygala tenuifolia (105)
12g [遠志]
Citrus reticulata (115) 10g [陳皮]
Glycyrrhiza uralensis (165)
20g [甘草]

Preparation

Have the herbs ground to fine powder. Simmer them in 1½ cups of honey over low flame for ½ hour, stirring regularly. Let cool. Ingest by the teaspoonful, 2-3 times a day, 5-7 days.

Remarks

The prescription helps to "transform phlegm" and facilitates coughing up excess of lodged phlegm. It forms a thick, viscous syrup which may be kept in a sealed jar for a long time. Use 5-7 days in a row to clean out lungs and bronchial tubes of accumulations of lodged phlegm. Highly recommended treatment for heavy smokers.

HANG-OVERS

Hovenia dulcis   20g [枳棋子]
Pueraria lobata (15) (roots)
10g [葛根粉]
Pueraria lobata (15) (flowers)
10g [葛花]

Preparation

Boil with 4 cups water in covered vessel until it decocts to 1½ cups, more or less. Strain. Take as 2 doses on empty stomach.

Tonics

IMPOTENCE

Cistanche salsa (169)   30g [肉蓯蓉]
Cuscuta japonica (172)
30g [菟絲子]
Schisandra chinensis (188)
30g [五味子]
Polygala tenuifolia (105)
30g [遠志]
Cnidium monnieri (173)
45g [蛇床子]

Preparation

Have the ingredients ground to a very fine powder. Then have them made into honey pills, or make the pills yourself by mixing the powders with enough honey to make a dough-like paste. Roll off small, round pellets between the thumb and fingers.
Take 10g of pills twice a day on empty stomach with some wine or liquor (no ice). Take twice daily for 2-3 months.

Remarks

While taking the medication, it is best to refrain from excess sexual activity. It is even better to practice Taoist retention techniques as part of the therapy.

Lycium chinense (183) 30g [枸杞子]
Schisandra chinensis (188)
　　　　　　　　30g [五味子]
Plantago asiatica (75) 30g [車前子]
Cuscuta japonica (172)
　　　　　　　　50g [菟絲子]
Rubus coreanus (194) 30g [覆盆子]

Preparation
Have the herbs made into honey pills, or make them yourself as above. Dosage same as above.

Cervus nippon (167) 100g [鹿茸]
Bombyx mori (silkworm)
　　　　　　　100g [原蠶蛾]

Preparation
Have the ingredients prepared, or prepare them yourself as above. Take 5 g of pills twice a day on empty stomach with wine or liquor (no ice). Take for 1 month.

Remarks
This is the strongest of the three tonic prescriptions given here for impotence. If over-stimulaton results, it can be neutralised by drinking cool tea.

PREMATURE EJACULATION

Nelumbo nucifera (stamens) (36)
　　　　　　100g [荷葉]
Euryale ferox (192)　100g [芡實]
Fossilised Bones of
Dinosaurs and Reptiles (102)
　　　　　　100g [龍骨]
Ostrea rivularis (103) 100g [牡蠣]
Rhus chinensis (190)　100g [五倍子]
Poria cocos (73)　100g [茯苓]

Preparation
Have the ingredients ground to a fine powder and mixed. Take 10 g with a large glass of hot water, twice a day (morning and night) on an empty stomach. Continue for 1 or 2 months.

Paratenodera sinensis (193)
　　　　　　10g [桑螵蛸]
Polygala tenuifolia (105)
　　　　　　5g [遠志]
Acorus gramineus (99) 5g [石菖蒲]
Fossilised bones of
dinosaurs and reptiles (102)
　　　　　　20g [龍骨]
Panax ginseng (159)　3g [人參]
Poria cocos (73)　10g [茯苓]
Angelica sinensis (178) 10g [當歸]

Chinemys reevesii (185)
　　　　　　15g [龜板]

Preparation
Boil with 5 cups water in covered vessel until it decocts to 1½ cups, more or less. Strain. Take as 2 doses per day on empty stomach. Continue for several weeks, or as necessary.

YANG SEN'S PRESCRIPTION FOR TONIC "SPRING WINE"

Cervus nippon (167)　150g [鹿茸]
Cervus nippon (glue) (167)
　　　　　　150g [鹿膠]
Equus asinus (glue) (179)
　　　　　　150g [阿膠]
Chinemys reevesii (glue) (185)
　　　　　　150g [龜膠]
Angelica sinensis (178) 60g [當歸]
Rehmannia glutinosa (176)
　　　　　　150g [熟地黃]
Astragalus membranaceus (161)
　　　　　　80g [黃耆]
Panax ginseng (best quality) (159)
　　　　　　20g [人參]
Rubus coreanus (194)　20g [覆盆子]
Lycium chinense (183) 60g [枸杞子]
Dried Human Placenta (166)
　　　　　　60g [胎盤]
Ligustrum japonicum (seeds)
　　　　　　60g [女貞子]
Cynomorium songaricum
　　　　　　60g [鎖陽]
gekko gecko (Red-Spotted Lizard)
　1 male and 1 female [蛤蚧]
Hippocampus kelloggi (Sea-Horse)
　2 or about 60g [海馬]

Preparation
Steep the ingredients in a large ceramic vessel with 6 litres of strong liquor, such as brandy, Chinese *gao liang*, vodka, etc. for 6 months or more. The vessel should be well sealed. After 6 months or so, pour off half the brew, and strain well through cheesecloth or filter paper. Refill the vessel with three fresh bottles of liquor, reseal, and steep for another 6 months or so. Use the entire batch the second time. The Spring Wine may be flavoured to taste with honey or sugar. To make a pleasing liqueur, add chopped chunks of rock crystal sugar to the strained liquor.

Dosage
Drink 1-2 ounces before retiring each night, more in winter, less in summer.

Remarks
We have it on good authority that this is Yang Sen's genuine personal prescription, developed by himself.

Chinese wolfberry stewed with beef

Herbal Recipes

Food is indispensible in daily life; but the art of deriving the most tonic effect from it is one which the Chinese have developed since antiquity by the application of their philosophy of balance to diet, and to match the diet to its tonifying effects on bodily functions. The use of tonics taken with food pre-date their use as medicine. Combined with food, tonics are absorbed better and are seen as a superior way to keep bodily functions in trim. Medicinal tonics, as the Chinese saying puts it, are inferior to food tonics.

The recipes that follow are a selection of herbal recipes which have earned their popularity both for their taste and their efficacy. They are well established in the treasurehouse of Chinese folk recipes. The herbal ingredients, if not common herbs, are readily obtainable at a Chinese herbalist, along with other herbs and herbal prescriptions mentioned earlier in this chapter. Herbal recipes and their place in the development of Chinese herbal medicine are discussed in Chapter 1.

Quantities given in the recipes serve 4—5 persons.

薏苡仁燉雞
PEARL BARLEY ("JOB'S TEARS") STEWED WITH CHICKEN (78)

Therapeutic benefits: Nutritive; tonic; diuretic; relieves arthritic pain in joints.

Ingredients:

1.2—1.4 kg (2.5—3lb)	chicken
310 g (10 oz)	fresh mushrooms, sliced
3—5	spring onions (scallions), finely chopped
3—5 slices	ginger-root, finely chopped
1	fresh orange, juiced
30 g (1 oz)	pearl barley *Coix lacryma-jobi* (78), ground, including husks.
To taste	salt, pepper and wine
10 cups (2½ litres)	water

Method:

Crush or coarsely grind the pearl barley, including husks.

Chop entire chicken into 2 cm (1 in) chunks, including bones, with a heavy cleaver. Wash well, place in a large stew-pot with 10 cups water.

Add crushed pearl barley, ginger, then bring to rolling boil, cover, lower heat, and simmer for 2 hours, or until chicken is tender.

For the very young, elderly or ailing patients, remove chicken to a separate dish, strain broth to remove barley pulp, then return chicken to the broth; otherwise, skip this step and leave pulp in the stew.

Add mushrooms, spring onions (scallions), salt and pepper to taste, a dash of wine, then reheat and serve.

淮山枸杞子燉牛展
CHINESE WOLFBERRY STEWED WITH BEEF (183)

Therapeutic benefits: Tonic for yang energy; aphrodisiac; promotes hormone secretions; enhances strength and endurance.

Ingredients:

500 g (1 lb)	beef tenderloin cut into 2 cm (1 in) cubes
60 g (2 oz)	butter
2	large carrots, cut into 1 cm (½ in) chunks
3	onions, sliced into crescents
1 cup (8 fl oz)	fresh green peas
1 cup (8 fl oz)	tomato sauce
30 g (1 oz)	Chinese wolfberry *Lycium chinense* (183)
3½ cups (28 fl oz)	water

Method:

Sprinkle cubed beef with salt and pepper.

Heat butter in a wok, add beef, and stir-fry until brown.

Add onions and stir-fry another 1—2 minutes.

Add tomato sauce, 3 cups water, Chinese wolfberry; cover, simmer for 2 hours.

Half an hour before done, add carrots and peas, salt and pepper to taste.

For thick broth, dissolve 2 teaspoons cornstarch in ½ cup water, and stir into stew 10 minutes before done.

Eat the herb together with beef and other ingredients.

海松子蛋湯
EGGS IN KOREAN PINE SEED BROTH

Therapeutic benefits: Tonic; nutritive; enhances strength and endurance.

Ingredients:

15 g (½ oz)	Korean pine seed *Pinus koraiensis*, crushed
6 cups (1½ litres)	water
5	chicken eggs
5	large dried black mushrooms, soaked and cut into strips
5	fresh spring onions (scallions), chopped small.
1 tablespoon	vinegar
To taste	salt, pepper and wine
500 g (1 lb)	chicken parts (for stock)

Method:

Boil pine seeds in 6 cups water, simmer until fluid is reduced to about 4 cups; strain through a cheesecloth, reserve broth, discard dregs.

Bring 3 cups water to boil with 1 tablespoon vinegar; break eggs one by one, and gently place in simmering water to poach about 1 minute; remove gently with a slotted spoon, rinse under cold water, and set aside.

Add chicken bones and parts to pine seed broth, boil for 30—60 minutes, strain out bones, reserve broth.

Bring chicken/pine seed broth to boil, add salt, pepper and wine to taste. Add mushrooms and spring onions (scallions). Gently place poached eggs in broth and simmer for 1 minute.

Place 1 egg and some mushroom into individual soup bowls, then ladle broth on top; serve.

當歸咖喱飯
ANGELICA CURRY RICE (178)

Therapeutic benefits: promotes blood circulation; improves complexion; enhances metabolism; tonifies yin energy.

Ingredients:

310 g (10 oz)	lean beef, or deboned chicken
3	onions, sliced into crescents
1	large carrot, cut into 1 cm (½ in) pieces
1	large potato, cut into 1 cm (½ in) pieces
1 cup (8 fl oz)	fresh green peas
1½ tablespoons	curry powder
2 tablespoons	flour
3 tablespoons	butter
To taste	salt and pepper
15 g (½ oz)	*Angelica sinensis*, thinly sliced (178)
5 cups (1¼ litres)	water

Method:

Boil sliced angelica in 2 cups water, until fluid is reduced by about half; set aside, do not discard pulp.

Cut beef or chicken into 2 cm (1 in) chunks.

Heat 1 tablespoon butter in a wok, add flour and stir well to thicken, then add curry powder, stir well to mix; then add 3 cups water, stir well to mix, then add carrots and potatoes, stir, cover, simmer on low heat.

In a separate wok or pan, heat 1 tablespoon butter, then stir-fry beef or chicken until just done. Remove to a plate.

Add another 1 tablespoon butter to wok and stir-fry onions until soft, remove and set aside.

When carrots and potatoes are done, add cooked meat and onions to the stew-pot and return to boil. Then add angelica broth with pulp, peas, return to boil and stir 1—2 minutes, add salt and pepper to taste.

Serve over rice or noodles.

何首烏鯉魚湯
POLYGONUM MULTIFLORUM AND CARP SOUP (177)

Therapeutic benefits: Tonic; stimulant; promotes hormone secretions.

Ingredients:

1	silver carp (trout, bream or snapper) about 30 cm (12 in) long
To taste	white pepper
To taste	chili oil and wine
15 g (½ oz)	*Polygonum multiflorum* (177)
8 cups (2 litres)	water

Method:

Bring herb to boil in 2 cups water, then simmer over low heat until reduced by about half; retain broth with pulp.

Gut the fish, but do not scale it; be careful not to break gall bladder and let bile run into the meat; rinse well under cold water; cut off the head, cut fish in half length-wise, then cut each half in half, making a total of 5 large pieces, including head.

Bring 6 cups water to boil, add 1—2 teaspoon salt, add the fish, simmer over low heat, covered, until scales and bones are tender, about 1½ hours.

When done, add herb broth and pulp to soup, return to boil, then remove from heat.

Season to taste with white pepper, chili oil, and wine. Serve.

茴香牛肉
FENNEL BEEF (96)

Thereapeutic benefits: Antitussive; expectorant; carminative; stomachic.

Ingredients:

410 g (13 oz)	beef tenderloin, cut into 2 cm (1 in) cubes
90 g (3 oz)	white sesame seeds
2 tablespoons	butter
To taste	soy sauce, sugar and wine
15 g (½ oz)	fennel *Foeniculum vulgare* (96)
1 cup (8 fl oz)	water

Method:

Stir-fry seasame seeds in dry wok until golden-brown, then crush to fine powder in mortar or food processor.

Roll cut beef in sesame seed powder until completely coated. Set aside for 1—2 hours.

Stir-fry fennel until fragrant, then grind to fine powder (or buy it ground from herbalist).

Heat 2 tablespoons butter in a wok until hot and add beef; stir-fry quickly 20—30 seconds, then add 1 cup water, bring to boil, season to taste with soy sauce, sugar, and wine; cover and simmer over low heat for 30 minutes.

Place beef and broth into a serving bowl, add ground fennel, stir well, and serve.

川芎蛤蜊湯
HEMLOCK PARSLEY ROOT AND CLAM SOUP (121)

Therapeutic benefits: sedative; analgesic; emmenogogue; warming to energy system in cold weather.

Ingredients:

310 g (10 oz)	clam (without shells)
3	carrots, diced in 2 cm (1 in) cubes
3	potatoes, diced in 2 cm (1 in) cubes
3	spring onions (scallions), minced
3 slices	ginger-root, minced
To taste	curry powder, salt and pepper

Pearl barley ("Jobs Tears") stewed with chicken

BROOMRAPE SEA FOOD HOT-POT (169)

Therapeutic benefits: tonic; aphrodisiac; restores physical strength; stimulates energy system.

Ingredients:
Prepare and cut following ingredients for hot-pot style dining:

500 g (1 lb)	Boneless white fish and boned (flounder, sole, tuna, etc)
310 g (10 oz)	clams or oysters, without shell
250 g (8 oz)	shrimp
1 head	cabbage
2	large carrots
6	spring onions (scallions)
185 g (6 oz)	fresh mushrooms
2 cakes	soft beancurd
8 cups (2 litres)	chicken or fish stock
15 g (½ oz)	broomrape *Cistanche salsa* (169), minced

Method:
Scale, skin, gut, and bone the fish, rinse well, cut into bite-size pieces; rinse clams in cold water; clean squid and cut into bite-size pieces; rinse shrimp and place on a plate; cut all other ingredients for the hot-pot and place each on separate plates.

Put minced herb in a large pot with stock, bring to boil, season to taste with salt, pepper and wine; then add half of fish and other ingredients, return to boil, then place on table on a portable burner, with remaining ingredients set on the table, to be added to the hot-pot as needed.

Consume the broth and herb pulp along with other ingredients, for maximum medicinal benefits.

"HORNY GOAT WEED" ASSORTED HOT-POT (168)

Therapeutic benefits: aphrodisiac; tonic; warming; enhances circulation; improves memory and other mental functions.

Ingredients:

410 g (13 oz)	calves liver, sliced

15 g (½ oz)	hemlock parsley root *Ligusticum wallichii* (121), sliced thinly
8 cups (2 litres)	water

Method:
Bring sliced herbs to boil in 3 cups water, simmer until fluid is reduced by about half; strain through cheesecloth, reserve broth, discard pulp.

Place carrots and potatoes in a pot, add herb broth, add 5 cups water, bring to boil, cover, simmer until cooked.

Wash clams with salted water, rinse well and add to the pot together with minced spring onions (scallions) and minced ginger; add salt and pepper to taste.

Return to boil, simmer 3—5 minutes, serve.

TUKAHOE AND MUSHROOM RICE (73)

Therapeutic benefits: sedative; diuretic; promotes hormone secretions.

Ingredients:

625 g (1¼ lb)	rice
15 g (½ oz)	dried black mushrooms
3 cakes	dried beancurd
1 cup (8 fl oz)	green peas
1 tablespoon	soy sauce
To taste	wine, salt and pepper
15 g (½ oz)	tukahoe *Poria cocos* (73)
310 g (10 oz)	rice

Method:
Soak herb in just enough water to cover it, for 1 hour, then mash to pulp.

Soak mushrooms in hot water, rinse clean, cut into thin strips; dice beancurd into bite-size cubes.

Wash rice and rinse, put in a pot or rice-cooker with sufficient water to cook it. Add 1 tablespoon soy sauce, a dash of wine, and salt and pepper to taste; stir.

Add herb pulp, sliced mushrooms, cubed beancurd; stir, cover, then cook as you normally cook rice, until all water is absorbed.

When done, add fresh green peas; stir gently to mix flavours, and serve.

1 dozen	fish balls, cut in half or
2 cakes	fish-paste cut into small chunks
2 cakes	soft beancurd
1 head	cabbage, cut in strips
2 bunches	spinach, cut in strips
6	spring onions (scallions)
To taste	salt, pepper, wine and vinegar
15 g (½ oz)	"Horny Goat Weed" *Epimedium sagittatum* (168)
2.25 l (4 quarts	chicken stock
3 cups (24 fl oz)	water

Method:

Bring herb leaves to boil in 3 cups water, cover and simmer until reduced to 1 cup. Strain through cheesecloth, reserve broth, discard pulp.

Prepare stock from chicken bones or seaweed, 2 quarts.

Bring stock to boil, add herb broth, add salt, pepper, wine and vinegar to taste; add half of ingredients, return to boil, immediately place on table on portable burner, and serve, adding remaining ingredients to pot as required during the meal.

CINNAMON CURRY RICE (92)

Therapeutic benefits: astringent; stomachic, tonic; stimulant, anagestic; relieves fatique; promotes circulation.

Ingredients:

250 g (8 oz)	lean pork, cut into bite-sized pieces
2	onions sliced into crescents
2	potatoes, cubed small
1	carrot, cubed small
1	large apple, minced
2 tablespoons	curry powder
2 tablespoons	flour
3 cloves	garlic, minced
4 cups (1 litre)	stock or water
4 tablespoons	butter
To taste	salt and pepper
310 g (10 oz)	rice
15 g (½ oz)	cinnamon *Cinnamomum cassia* (92)
300 g (10 oz)	rice

| 2-3 cups | water (16—24 fl oz) |
| 2 tablespoons | frying oil |

Method:

Bring cinnamon to boil in 2 cups water, simmer covered until reduced to 1 cup; strain, discard pulp, reserve broth.

Cook enough rice for 5 persons.

Heat butter in a wok, add flour and stir well to mix and thicken; then add curry powder and stir well to mix; then add a little stock or water and mix well; return to boil, add carrot, potatoes, and apple, cover, simmer on low heat.

In a separate wok or pan, stir-fry sliced pork quickly in a little oil along with garlic. Remove and reserve.

When carrots and potatoes are almost done, add cinnamon broth, pork and onions to the pot, return to boil, simmer for a few minutes, then serve over rice.

SAFFLOWER STEWED WITH BEEF (123)

Therapeutic benefits: uterine astringent in dysmenorrhea; tonic nutrient after childbirth.

Serves 5 persons

Ingredients:

500 g (1 lb)	beef tenderloin
2	carrots, cubed
5	potatoes, cubed

Gastrodia elata mixed rice

1	onion, sliced into crescents
250 g (8 oz)	fresh mushrooms, sliced
1 cup (8 fl oz)	green peas
½ cup (4 fl oz)	tomato juice
2 tablespoons	butter
2 tablespoons	flour
To taste	salt pepper and soy sauce
15 g (½ oz)	Safflower *Carthamus tinctorius* (123)
5 cups (1¼ litres)	water

Method:

Put 5 cups water in a large stew-pot and bring to boil.

Cut beef tenderloin in half (2 large pieces) and place in boiling water together with safflower and cubed carrots.

In a separate wok or pan, heat butter, then add flour and stir well to thicken; add tomato juice and mix well, then remove and reserve.

When potatoes are almost done, remove beef from the broth, add butter/flour/tomato mix to the stew-pot, stir well to thicken; add salt, pepper, and soy sauce to taste.

Cut cooked beef into bite-size chunks, return to stew-pot, bring back to boil, then add mushrooms, peas; simmer 3—4 minutes more, and serve.

This is a very fortifying dish; be sure to consume broth and safflower for maximum medicinal benefits.

天麻什錦飯
GASTRODIA ELATA MIXED RICE (109)

Therapeutic benefits: tonic for headaches and rheumatism; stimulant for nervous disorders; improves mental functions.

Ingredients:
310 g (10 oz)	rice
90 g (3 oz)	chicken meat, boned and skinned, cut into small chunks
1	large fresh bamboo shoot (or 1 small can), sliced thin
1	large carrot, sliced thin

5	dried black mushrooms, soaked in hot water, sliced thinly
1 cup (8 fl oz)	green peas
To taste	salt, pepper and soy sauce
15 g (½ oz)	*Gastrodia elata*
1½ cups (12 fl oz)	water

Method:

Soak the herb in 1½ cups water for 1 hour to soften; then add it and its water to rice pot with the rice.

Add all above ingredients to the rice pot, season to taste with salt, pepper, and soy sauce; stir well to mix ingredients, then cook as you normally cook rice.

When done, add the green peas, stir gently to mix, and serve.

山藥魚片湯
CHINESE YAM AND FISH SOUP (163)

Therapeutic benefits: nutritive; tonic; digestant; controls nocturnal emission of semen, incontinence of urine, and night sweats.

Ingredients:
410 g (13 oz)	any type of white fish, skinned and boned, sliced to bite-size pieces
150 g (5 oz)	white turnip, finely shredded
150 g (5 oz)	miso paste
1 large sheet	dried seaweed, cut into strips
To taste	pepper, minced scallion
15 g (½ oz)	Chinese yam *Dioscorea opposita* (163), mashed to a paste
3	spring onions (scallions), minced
3 cups (24 fl oz)	water

Method:

Bring 3 cups water to boil, add seaweed, boil for 3 minutes, then remove seaweed pulp with a slotted spoon.

Add mashed yam, sliced fish and shredded turnip to the broth, return to boil, cover, then simmer over low heat for 5 minutes.

Sprinkle some pepper and minced scallion into individual soup bowls, then ladle servings of soup and solid ingredients into each bowl, stir, and serve.

當歸火鍋
ANGELICA HOT-POT (178)

Therapeutic benefits: promotes blood circulation; stimulates metabolism; tonifies yin energy.

Ingredients:
410 g (13 oz)	any type white fish meat, boned and skinned, sliced into bite size pieces
3 cakes	soft beancurd, cut to bite-sized cubes
1 head	cabbage, cut into strips for hot-pot
5	large dried black mushrooms, soaked in hot water, cut into thin strips
5 cups (1¼ litres)	chicken stock
To taste	salt, pepper and soy suace
15 g (½ oz)	*Angelica sinensis* (178), sliced thin

Method:

Bring chicken stock to boil, add sliced angelica, simmer for 20 minutes.

Add fish, beancurd, mushrooms to soup, return to boil, then add cabbage, and simmer until tender (about 5 minutes).

Set on table on a portable burner and serve.

杜仲鹹魚湯
EUCOMMIA BARK AND SMOKED SALMON SOUP (175)

Therapeutic benefits: tonic; sedative; analgesic; improves nervous functions.

Ingredients:
410 g (13 oz)	smoked salmon (or salt-fish), sliced into bite-size pieces
150 g (5 oz)	white turnip, finely shredded
2 cakes	soft beancurd, cut into small cubes
150 g (5 oz)	miso paste

5 g (1/6 oz)	*Eucommia ulmoides* (175)
6 cups (1½ litres)	water
A sprinkling	pepper, minced scallion

Method:

Bring herb to boil in 2 cups water, cover, simmer until liquid is reduced by about half; strain broth and reserve, discard pulp.

Bring 4 cups water to boil, add miso, stir well.

Add sliced fish and shredded turnip and beancurd to the soup, then add herb broth; adjust salinity by adding more salt or more plain water, to taste; return to boil, simmer 6—7 minutes.

Sprinkle some pepper and minced spring onions (scallions) into individual soup bowls, ladle servings of soup and solid ingredients on top, stir, and serve.

女貞子火鍋
"WAX PRIVET SEED" HOT POT

Therapeutic benefits: nutritive; tonic; stimulant to nervous system.

Ingredients:
500 g (1 lb)	beef liver (or chicken livers) cut into bite-sized pieces
90 g (3 oz)	fresh mushrooms, sliced
5	large black dried mushrooms
1	large carrot, sliced thinly
1 packet	bean-flour thread-noodles
1 head	cabbage
1—2 bunches	spinach
5 cups (1¼ litres)	chicken, beef, or pork stock
To taste	salt, pepper, wine and soy sauce
15 g (½ oz)	wax privet seed *Ligustrum lucidum*
3 cups (24 fl oz)	water

Method:

Soak dried mushrooms in hot water, then slice into thin strips; soak thread-noodles in cold water until soft, then set aside to drain; wash spinach and cabbage and cut in strips for the hot-pot.

Bring herb seeds to boil in 3 cups water, cover, simmer until reduced to 1 cup, strain, reserve broth, discard pulp.

Bring stock to boil, add carrots, simmer; when carrots are soft, add both varieties of mushroom, add herb broth, then season to taste with salt, pepper, wine, and soy sauce.

Return to boil, add half of liver, bean threads, cabbage, and spinach, simmer 2—3 minutes, then transfer to a portable burner on table. Place remaining ingredients on the table on plates and add to the hot-pot as required.

人參鯛魚湯
GINSENG AND PORGY FISH HEAD SOUP (159)

Therapeutic benefits: tonic; stimulant; aphrodisiac; stomachic; promotes harmone secretions; retards aging.

Ingredients:
1 medium size	Porgy or bream fish head *Pagrosomus major*
To taste	salt, pepper, wine and vinegar
2	minced spring onions (scallions)
15 g (½ oz)	ginseng *Panax ginseng* (any variety) (159), sliced thinly
2-3 drops	sesame oil
8 cups (2 litres)	water

Method:

Cut fish head in half, then cut each half into 2 or 3 large chunks (this is a hard-headed fish, so it is best to have your fishmonger chop it for you).

Coat fish head chunks well with salt and set aside to marinate for 30 minutes.

Blanch salted fish head briefly in boiling water, remove quickly, and rinse clean under cold running water.

Bring sliced ginseng to boil in 3 cups water; simmer about 1 hour, or until fluid is reduced by about half; strain, reserve both pulp and broth, separately.

Add 5 cups water to ginseng broth and bring to boil in a large pot; add fish head chunks and return to boil; remove scum that rises to the surface, then season to taste with salt, wine,

add dash of vinegar; cover and simmer over low heat for 10 minutes.

Sprinkle some pepper and minced spring onions (scallions) into individual soup bowls, add 2—3 drops sesame oil, some of the ginseng pulp, then ladle soup and fish on top, stir, and serve. (Ginseng pulp will be soft enough to eat and it tastes good; it retains some medicinal properties even after broth is extracted, and should be consumed.)

人參蒸鷄腿
GINSENG STEAMED WITH CHICKEN LEGS (159)

Therapeutic benefits: tonic; stimulant; aphrodisiac; promotes hormone secretions; retards aging.

Ingredients:
3 large or 4 small	chicken legs
1 cup (8 fl oz)	rice wine or dry sherry
To taste	white pepper
2	spring onions (scallions), minced
5 slices	ginger root
15 g (½ oz)	ginseng *Panax ginseng* (159) (any variety), thinly sliced

Method:

Cut each chicken leg in half at the joint; with a heavy cleaver chop each half into 2 pieces, including bone.

Place chicken chunks in a Pyrex or ceramic bowl, add sliced ginseng and ginger, add wine or sherry.

Place bowl in a steamer basket or steamer-wok, and steam over high heat for 1 hour.

Sprinkle pepper and minced spring onions (scallions) into individual soup bowls, then ladle chicken chunks, ginseng pulp, and broth into soup bowls, stir, and serve.

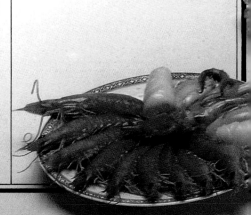

芡實餃子
FOXNUT DUMPLINGS (192)

Therapeutic benefits: tonic; analgesic; astringent in spermatorrhea; enhances strength and energy.

Ingredients:

185 g (6 oz)	ground pork
2	onions, well minced
1 cup (8 fl oz)	tender baby green peas
20-25	thin-skin dumpling wrappers*
To taste	salt, pepper, white wine, soy sauce and sesame oil
15 g (½ oz)	foxnut *Euryale ferox* (192)
3 l (3 quarts)	water
3 tablespoons	frying oil

Method:

Crush the herb and soak in water for one hour; strain, discard water, reserve herb.

Put ground pork in bowl, add minced onions and tender peas and mix; season to taste with salt, pepper, wine, soy sauce, sesame oil, and mix well.

Add crushed, softened herb and mix well.

Wrap stuffing mix into individual dumpling-skins, seal edges, and set on a floured tray.

To make boiled dumplings: bring 3 litres water to rolling boil; drop about 20 dumplings into the water; when it returns to boil, add ¾ cup cold water; when it returns to boil again, add ¾ cup cold water. After adding the third dose of cold water and returning to boil, scoop out the dumplings with slotted spoon and serve immediately.

To make "pot-stickers:" in large flat skillet heat enough oil to coat the entire skillet; place dumplings one by one into the skillet; when the skillet is full and dumplings are frying, quickly pour ½ cup tepid water into the skillet and quickly cover; allow to steam and sizzle for 3—5 minutes, then remove and serve.

Serve dumplings with saucers of soy sauce, vinegar, sesame oil, and chili sauce, as condiments.

* available in Chinese groceries and most large super-markets, Oriental foods section).

牛膝魚丸湯
ACHYRANTHES BIDENTATA AND FISH-BALL SOUP (124)

Therapeutic benefits: detoxifies blood; diurectic; emmenogogue; tonic; stimulates energy channels.

Ingredients:

310 g (10 oz)	any type of mild white fish meat, boned and skinned
1	egg
1½ teaspoon	cornstarch
½	white turnip, shredded
125 g (4 oz)	spinach, cut for soup
125 g (4 oz)	clams and/or shrimp (optional)
15 g (½ oz)	*Achyranthes bidentata* (124)
7 cups (1¾ fl oz)	water

Method:

Bring herb to boil in 2 cups water, simmer and reduce by half, about 1 hour; strain, reserve broth, discard pulp.

Dice fish meat, then mince it very well with a knife or mincing tool; place mashed fish into a bowl, beat the egg separately, then stir into fish; dissolve 1½ teaspoon cornstarch in ¼ cup cold water, add to fish mix, and stir well with fingers or a spoon.

Bring·5 cups water to rolling boil in a large pot; use a small spoon to transfer lumps of fish-paste mix one by one into boiling water; as fish-balls cook and float to the surface, remove them to a bowl with slotted spoon. Continue until all fish-paste is cooked and fish-balls are removed to a bowl.

Add turnip, spinach, clams and/or shrimp to soup, season to taste with salt, pepper, and soy sauce; then add herb broth; when soup returns to boil, return the cooked fish-balls to the soup, simmer for 2—3 minutes more, remove from heat and serve.

Broomrape sea food hot-pot

Bibliography

A Barefoot Doctor's Manual. (Contemporary Chinese Paramedical Manual). Philadelphia: Running Press, 1977.

Chang, Jolan. *The Tao of Love and Sex.* London: Granada, 1979.

Chinese Medicinal Herbs. Compiled by Li Shih chen. San Francisco: Georgetown Press, 1973.

Gulik, R.H. van. *Sexual Life in Ancient China.* Lieden: E.J. Brill; Atlantic Highlands, N.J: Humanities Press, 1961.

Keys, John D. *Chinese Herbs.* Tokyo: Charles E Tuttle, 1976.

Lin Yutang. *The Wisdom of China.* London: Michael Joseph; New York: Modern Library, 1974.

Mann, Dr Felix. *Acupuncture: The Chinese Art of Healing. 3rd Ed.* London: William Heinemann Medical Books, 1978.
— *The Treatment of Disease by Acupuncture.* London: William Heinemann Medical Books, 1964 (reprinted 1980).
— *The Meridians of Acupuncture.* London: William Heinemann Medical Books, 1954 (reprinted 1973).
— *Atlas of Acupuncture.* London: William Heinemann Medical Books, 1966.

Needham, Joseph. *Science and Civilization in China,* (7 volumes). Cambridge: Cambridge University Press, 1954.

Palos, Stephen. *The Chinese Art of Healing.* New York: McGraw Hill, 1971; New York: Bantam Books, 1972.

Read, Bernard E. *Chinese Materia Medica:* vol 1, *Dragon and Snake Drugs,* (1934), vol. 2, *Fish Drugs,* (1939), vol. 3, *Insect Drugs,* (1941). Reprinted in Taipei (3 vols in 1): Southern Materials Press, 1977.
— *Chinese Materia Medica: Turtle and Shellfish Drugs,*(1937), *Avian Drugs,* (1932), *Turtle and Shellfish Drugs* (1937), *A Compendium of Minerals and Stones,* (1936), Reprinted in Taipei (3 vols in 1): Southern Materials Press, 1976.
— *Chinese Materia Medica: Animal Drugs,* (1931). Reprinted in Taipei: Southern Materials Press,1976.

Said, Hakim Mohammed. *Medicine in China.* Karachi: Hamdard Foundation, 1981.

Stuart, Rev. G.A. *Chinese Materia Medica: Vegetable Kingdom.* Shanghai: American Presbeterian Press, 1911. Reprinted in Taipei: Southern Materials Centre, 1976.

Veith, Ilza. *Huang Ti Nei Ching Su Wen, The Yellow Emperor's Classic of Internal Medicine, New Edition.* Berkeley: University of California Press, 1972.

Wong, K.C. and Wu, L.T. *History of Chinese Medicine.* Shanghai: National Quarantine Service, 1936. Reprinted in Taipei: Southern Materials Centre, 1976.

Index

Herbs listed under their botanical names. Numbers refer to the order of listing commencing on page 81

Achyranthes bidentata (124)
Aconitum carmichaeli (91)
Acorus gramineus (99)
Adenophora tetraphylla (181)
Agastache rugosa (68)
Agkistrodon acutus (90)
Agrimonia pilosa (128)
Akebia quinata (76)
Alisma plantago aquatica (74)
Allium fistulosum (9)
Allium sativum (200)
Aloe barbadensis (22)
Alpinia oxyphylla (170)
Amomum xanthioides (72)
Anemarrhena asphodeloides (30)
Angelica anomala (7)
Angelica pubescens (83)
Angelica sinensis (178)
Apis mellifera (25)
Arctium lappa (12)
Areca catechu (197)
Arisaema consanguineum (142)
Aristolochia debilis (153)
Artemisia annua (66)
Artemisia capillaris (77)
Artemisia vulgaris (130)
Asarum sieboldii (6)
Aster tataricus (156)
Astragalus membranaceus (161)
Atractylodes chinensis (70)
Atractylodes macrocephala (162)
Belamcanda chinensis (51)
Bletilla striata (129)
Bos taurus domesticus or Bubalus bubalis (41)
Boswellia carterii (126)
Brucea javanica (57)
Bupleurum falcatum (16)
Buthus martensi (113)
Canarium album (54)
Cannabis sativa (23)
Carthamus tinctorius (123)
Cassia angustifolia (21)
Cassia tora (37)
Celosia argentea (35)
Cervus nippon (167)
Chaenomeles lagenaria (86)
Chinemys reevesii (185)
Chrysanthemum morifolium (14)
Cinnamomum cassia (92)
Cinnamomum cassia (2)
Cirsium japonicum (131)
Cistanche salsa (169)
Citrus reticulata (115)
Clematis chinensis (88)
Clerodendrum trichotomum (84)
Cnidium monnieri (173)
Codonopsis tangshen (160)
Coix lacryma jobi (78)
Coptis sinensis (59)
Cornus officinalis (187)
Crataegus pinnatifida (138)
Croton tiglium (28)
Cryptotympana pustulata (18)
Cucurbita moschata (198)
Curcuma aromatica (127)
Cuscuta japonica (172)
Cynanchum atratum (67)
Cynanchum stauntoni (146)
Cyperus rotundus (118)
Datura metel (158)
Dioscorea hypoglauca (80)
Dioscorea opposita (163)
Diospyros kaki (119)

Dipsacus asper (174)
Dried human placenta (166)
Dryobalanops aromatica (97)
Dryopteris crassirhizoma (199)
Eclipta prostrata (184)
Eleutherococcus gracilistylus (87)
Elsholtzia splendens (8)
Ephedra sinica (1)
Epimedium sagittatum (168)
Equus asinus (179)
Eriobotrya japonica (154)
Eucommia ulmoides (175)
Euodia rutaecarpa (94)
Eupatorium fortunei (69)
Euphorbia kansui (26)
Euphoria longan (180)
Euryale ferox (192)
Ferrosoferric oxide (101)
Foeniculum vulgare (96)
Forsythia suspensa (48)
Fossilised bones of dinosaurs and reptiles (102)
Fraxinus bungeana (63)
Fritillaria verticillata (147)
Gallus gallus domesticus (139)
Gardenia jasminoides (31)
Gastrodia elata (109)
Gentiana macrophylla (85)
Gentiana scabra (62)
Glycine max (17)
Glycyrrhiza uralensis (165)
Gypsum fibrosum (29)
Haliotis gigantea (108)
Hematite (111)
Hordeum vulgare (140)
Hydrous magnesium silicate (81)
Imperata cylindrica (46)
Inula britannica (145)
Isatis tinctoria (44)
Ledebouriella seseloides (5)
Lepidium apetalum (150)
Ligusticum wallichii (121)
Liriope spicata (182)
Lithospermum erythrorhizon (39)
Lonicera japonica (47)
Luffa cylindrica (89)
Lycium chinense (183)
Lycium chinense (65)
Lycoperdon perlatum (53)
Magnolia liliflora (11)
Magnolia officinalis (71)
Malva verticillata (82)
Manis pentadactyla (125)
Mentha arvensis (10)
Mirabilite (20)
Morus alba (13)
Moschus moschiferus (98)
Nelumbo nucifera (36)
Ostrea rivularis (103)
Paeonia lactiflora (43)
Paeonia moutan (42)
Panax ginseng (159)
Panax notoginseng (137)
Papaver somniferum (191)
Paratenodera sinensis (193)
Perilla frutescens (143)
Perilla frutescens (3)
Peucedanum decursivum (148)
Pharbitis nil (27)
Phellodendron amurense (61)
Pheretima aspergillum (112)
Phragmites communis (32)
Phyllostachys (33)
Pinellia ternata (141)
Plantago asiatica (75)
Platycodon grandiflorum (144)
Polygala tenuifolia (105)
Polygonum multiflorum (177)
Poncirus trifoliata (116)
Poria cocos (73)

Portulaca oleracea (56)
Prunella vulgaris (34)
Prunus armeniaca (152)
Prunus japonica (24)
Prunus persica (122)
Pueraria lobata (15)
Pulsatilla chinensis (55)
Quisqualis indica (196)
Red mercuric sulfide (100)
Rehmannia glutinosa (176)
Rehmannia glutinosa (38)
Rheum officinale (19)
Rhinoceros unicornis (40)
Rhus chinensis (190)
Rubia cordifolia (135)
Rubus coreanus (194)
Saiga tatarica (107)
Salvia miltiorrhiza (120)
Sanguisorba officinalis (134)
Sargassum fusiforme (151)
Saussurea lappa (117)
Schisandra chinensis (188)
Schizonepeta tenuifolia (4)
Scolopendra subspinipes (114)
Scrophularia ningpoensis (45)
Scutellaria baicalensis (60)
Scutellaria barbata (58)
Sepia esculenta (195)
Sophora flavescens (64)
Sophora japonica (133)
Sophora subprostrata (52)
Stemona tuberosa (157)
Syzygium aromaticum (95)
Taraxacum officinale (49)
Terminalia chebula (189)
Thuja orientalis (132)
Tribulus terrestris (171)
Trichosanthes kirilowii (149)
Trionyx sinensis (186)
Triticum aestivum (106)
Tussilago farfara (155)
Typha latifolia (136)
Uncaria rhynchophylla (110)
Viola yedoensis (50)
Zea mays (79)
Zingiber officinale (93)
Ziziphus jujuba (164)
Ziziphus jujuba (104)